The
HANDBOOK
of inequality and
socioeconomic
position

Mary Shaw, Bruna Galobardes, Debbie A. Lawlor,

John Lynch, Ben Wheeler and

George Davey Smith

For Lily Florence Wells

First published in Great Britain in 2007 by

The Policy Press
Fourth Floor, Beacon House
Queen's Road
Bristol BS8 1QU
UK

Tel no   +44 (0)117 331 4054
Fax no   +44 (0)117 331 4093
Email   tpp-info@bristol.ac.uk
www.policypress.org.uk

© Mary Shaw, Bruna Galobardes, Debbie A. Lawlor, John Lynch, Ben Wheeler and George Davey Smith 2007

ISBN 978 1 86134 766 4 paperback
ISBN 978 1 86134 767 1 hardback

British Library Cataloguing in Publication Data
A catalogue record for this book is available from the British Library.

Library of Congress Cataloging-in-Publication Data
A catalog record for this book has been requested.

Cover design by Qube Design Associates, Bristol
Front cover illustration kindly supplied by Steven Appleby
Printed in Great Britain by Hobbs the Printers, Southampton

WAYS TO MEASURE SOCIOECONOMIC POSITION.

i - HEIGHT:
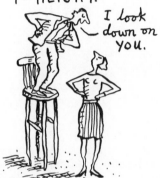
I look down on YOU.

ii - SHOE SIZE:
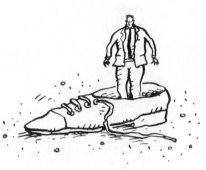

iii - VELOCITY OF BACK-SLAPPING:
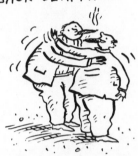

iv - DENSITY OF GLOOM:
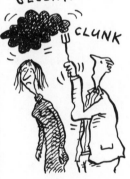
CLUNK

v - HEIGHT OF HOPPING & SKIPPING:
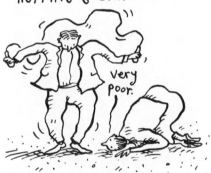
Very poor.

vi - QUANTITY OF SMILES:
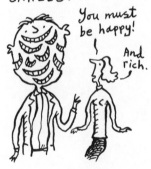
You must be happy!
And rich.

vii - CAKE:
I've had my cake AND eaten it.
None for YOU.
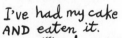
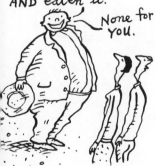

viii - NUMBER OF TELEVISION CHANNELS:
And number of televisions!
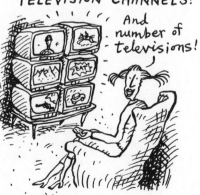

ix - NUMBER OF SOCIOECONOMIC STUDIES DONE ABOUT YOU:
Wow!
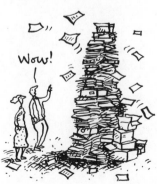

Table of contents by category

Part Three: Measures of inequality

Part Four: Theoretical and methodological issues

Table of contents by alphabetical order

Acknowledgements

Thanks to Dave Worth and all the team at Policy Press for their hard work and support throughout the process of producing this book. Thanks also to Dawn Rushen. Thanks to Steven Appleby for the wonderful cartoons. Census and geographical boundary data are Crown Copyright, and were obtained through ESRC/JISC agreements. Mary Shaw is funded by the South West Public Health Observatory.

How to use this book

This book is a toolbox for describing and assessing outcomes according to socioeconomic position (SEP). It is an extension of previous work published by the authors (Galobardes et al, 2006a, 2006b, 2006c, 2007). The book is designed to be of use to anyone researching or studying socioeconomic inequalities, including academics, policy makers, public health trainees and analysts and those working in local authorities. We have used examples from health inequalities research to explain the measures and methods we describe, but the book will have application beyond that area and should be of use to all those whose work involves the description and analysis of inequalities.

We use the term 'socioeconomic position' as an umbrella term to refer to the social and economic factors that influence what positions individuals or groups hold within society. We advocate using this as a generic term when referring to general issues of societal inequalities, and careful use of the more specific terms it covers.

For ease of use we have categorised the entries in the book. We highlight first some **key concepts** that are relevant to this topic area, such as deprivation, inequality and inequity. We then present a comprehensive collection of a range of **measures of socioeconomic position**, such as education, income and housing tenure. Note that some entries – such as poverty – appear both as key concepts and, in their operationalised versions, as measures. We then include various techniques for measuring the extent of inequalities. These **measures of inequality** include simple descriptive techniques such as absolute and relative differences as well as some more statistically complex measures such as the Gini coefficient and the Dissimilarity Index. Finally, we cover a few generic epidemiological concepts that may be helpful in the interpretation of inequalities, such as incidence, the ecological fallacy and lay epidemiology, which we have termed **theoretical and methodological issues**.

Where appropriate we have covered the strengths and limitations of particular measures of SEP and measures of inequality to guide people in their understanding and use of these. The question of which measure of SEP is best, however, will depend on the research question being posed. We hope that this book will assist people in understanding and using measures of SEP and in assessing the extent of socioeconomic inequalities.

References

Galobardes, B., Lynch, J. and Davey Smith, G. (2007) 'Measuring socioeconomic position in health research', *British Medical Bulletin*.

Galobardes, B., Shaw, M., Lawlor, D., Lynch, J. and Davey Smith, G. (2006a) 'Glossary: indicators of socioeconomic position (Part 1)', *Journal of Epidemiology and Community Health*, vol 60, pp 7-12.

Galobardes, B., Shaw, M., Lawlor, D., Lynch, J. and Davey Smith, G. (2006b) 'Glossary: indicators of socioeconomic position (Part 2)', *Journal of Epidemiology and Community Health*, vol 60, pp 95-101.

Galobardes, B., Shaw, M., Lawlor, D., Davey Smith, G. and Lynch, J. (2006c) 'Indicators of socioeconomic position', in J.M. Oakes and J. Kaufman (eds) *Methods in social epidemiology*, San Francisco, CA: Jossey-Bass.

Part One
Key concepts

1.1 Deprivation

'Deprivation' (often used in conjunction or interchangeably with the term 'disadvantage') is a term that refers to a variety of conditions experienced by people who lack certain resources in relation to others in the community, thereby making them 'deprived' compared to others in the population. 'Relative deprivation' can only occur in comparison with the condition of others. These conditions may be material, such as dietary intake, home environment, housing and clothing. Alternatively, they might be social conditions, referring to the rights of employment, community integration, recreation, education and so on. Several area-based indices of deprivation exist, differing in the components that are included and methods used. Numerous studies have reported an association between social and material deprivation and poor health outcomes.

Discussion point

In a rich society, no one should be allowed to suffer from deprivation such as homelessness, starvation and illness. This ideal is essential, not simply as a matter of human good, but as the price we pay for a measure of domestic tranquillity. (J.K. Galbraith, www.inequality.org)

... socio-economic deprivation includes a whole constellation of closely interrelated factors, such as lack of money, overcrowded and substandard housing, living in a poor locality, worse education, unsatisfying work or actual unemployment, and reduced social approval and self-esteem. (Rose, 1992, p 127)

References
Rose, G. (1992) *The strategy of preventive medicine*, Oxford: Oxford University Press.

Further reading
Gibbons, S., Green, A., Gregg, P. and Machin, S. (2005) 'Is Britain pulling apart? Area disparities in employment, education and crime', in N. Pearce and W. Paxton (eds) *Social justice: Building a fairer Britain*, London: Politico's Publishing, pp 219-39.
Townsend, P., Phillimore, P. and Beattie, A. (1988) *Health and deprivation: Inequality and the North*, London: Croom Helm.

See also: 1.10 Poverty; 1.15 Social exclusion; 2.8 Deprivation indices

1.2 Ethnicity

'Ethnicity' derives from the Greek word 'ethnos' and means 'nation' or 'people'. An ethnic group is now generally considered to be a community who share a number of characteristics, for example, some, but not necessarily all, of language, history, religion, geographical origin, mythologies, traditions and political system. The term is often linked to identity, in the formulation 'ethnic identity', and relates to the reporting of the experience of group membership. It is also often linked to the concept of minority status as in 'ethnic minorities', indicating people who live in a country that is not generally their land of family origin and in which they are not the majority population. These extended definitions are of course not automatically linked, and the majority population in a country has an ethnic identity.

Ethnicity is not a measure of socioeconomic position (SEP), but in some contexts, particularly within the US, it has been used as a proxy measure of SEP. In the US a portmanteau term 'race/ethnicity' is sometimes used, reflecting a notion of difference that extends beyond that of identity alone. In the US the use of ethnicity as an index of SEP is, in part, due to the historical relative absence of socioeconomic data in routine data sources in that country. For example, in a US Department of Health and Human Services report entitled *Health status of the disadvantaged*, a high proportion of tables present health indicators by what is referred to as 'race' and not by any explicitly socioeconomic measure (US DHHS, 1990).

The use of ethnicity in this way is clearly problematic. First, it can lead to the ignoring of socioeconomic differences in health status within minority ethnic populations. Indeed, until relatively recently the association between SEP and mortality among minority ethnic groups was little examined. Second, the use of ethnicity as a proxy for SEP often makes the inappropriate assumption that all members of minority ethnic groups are economically disadvantaged or deprived, an implied identity that, understandably, many people would want to reject. Third, it assumes that common interests are shared within but not between ethnic groups, whereas the real interests of the working class, for example, may be shared across ethnic groups more than the interests of an ethnic group are shared by the capitalist and working-class members within that group. Finally, this approach has difficulty accounting for cases in which minority ethnic groups who are economically disadvantaged compared with the majority population have better health outcomes – for example, the low mortality of Hispanic adults in the US (Sorlie et al, 1993) and of African

Caribbean men in Britain (Davey Smith et al, 2000) and the low postneonatal mortality among offspring of women of Bangladeshi or Indian origin in Britain (Raleigh and Balarajan, 1995).

In health studies ethnic group differences are frequently the topic of enquiry, with attempts being made to understand the contribution of socioeconomic circumstances to such differences. This is problematic because socioeconomic measures may have a different meaning in different ethnic groups and not indicate material circumstances in the same manner. Thus, at the same level of income in the US Black households have considerably lower wealth than White households (Blau and Graham, 1990); within the same jobs, Blacks have greater levels of exposure than Whites to work-related hazards (Robinson, 1984); education brings lower returns in terms of income, occupational status, and avoidance of unemployment among Blacks than among Whites (Hacker, 1995); and the purchasing power of Blacks is less than that of Whites at a given income level with respect to food, housing and other necessary expenditures (Williams and Collins, 1995). At a given level of income, occupational position, or educational achievement, Blacks are disadvantaged in other domains with respect to Whites, and adjustment for these factors will not fully adjust for differences in socioeconomic circumstances between the groups.

A similar situation pertains in Britain. For example, housing tenure is not an adequate marker of housing quality, since South Asian owner-occupiers are at increased likelihood of being in accommodation that is older, unmodernised, and overcrowded (Jones, 1993) or lacking in basic amenities (Nazroo, 1997). This is important because often studies of ethnic group differences in health status statistically adjust for socioeconomic measures and then suggest that any residual effects are due to genes, culture or behaviours, whereas they may reflect inadequate adjustment for commensurate measures of SEP. Minority ethnic group members may also suffer from the effects of discrimination and racism within the societies in which they live (Krieger, 1999), which itself may have health effects over and above differential socioeconomic circumstances.

References

Blau, F. and Graham J. (1990) 'Black-white differences in wealth and asset composition', *Quarterly Journal of Economics*, vol 105, pp 321-9.

Davey Smith, G., Chaturvedi, N., Harding, S., Nazroo, J. and Williams R. (2000) 'Ethnic inequalities in health: a review of UK epidemiological evidence', *Critical Public Health*, vol 10, pp 375-408.

Hacker, A. (1995) *Two nations: Black and white, separate, hostile, unequal*, New York, NY: Ballantine Books.

Jones, T. (1993) *Britain's ethnic minorities*, London: Policy Studies Institute.

Krieger, N. (1999) 'Embodying inequality: a review of concepts, measures, and methods for studying health consequences of discrimination', *International Journal of Health Services*, vol 29, pp 295-352.

Nazroo, J. (1997) *The health of Britain's ethnic minorities: Findings from a national survey*, London: Policy Studies Institute.

Raleigh, V. and Balarajan, R. (1995) 'The health of infants and children among ethnic minorities', in B. Botting (ed) *The health of our children*, London: HMSO, OPCS Series DS, vol II, pp 82-94.

Robinson, J. (1984) 'Racial inequality and the probability of occupational-related injury or illness', *Milbank Memorial Fund Quarterly*, vol 62, pp 567-90.

Sorlie, P., Backlund, E., Johnson, N. and Rogot, E. (1993) 'Mortality by Hispanic status in the United States', *Journal of the American Medical Association*, vol 270, pp 2464-8.

US DHHS (United States Department of Health and Human Services) (1990) *US DHSS Chartbook. Health status of the disadvantaged*, Washington, DC: US DHHS.

Williams, D. and Collins, C. (1995) 'US socioeconomic and racial differences in health: patterns and explanations', *Annual Review of Sociology*, vol 21, pp 349-86.

Further reading

Davey Smith, G. (2000) 'Learning to live with complexity: ethnicity, socioeconomic position, and health in Britain and the United States', *American Journal of Public Health*, vol 90, pp 1694-8.

Krieger, N. (2005) 'Stormy weather: race, gene expression, and the science of health disparities', *American Journal of Public Health*, vol 95, pp 2155-60.

Nazroo, J. (1998) 'Genetic, cultural or socio-economic vulnerability? Explaining ethnic inequalities in health', in M. Bartley, D. Blane and G. Davey Smith (eds) *The sociology of health inequalities*, Oxford: Blackwell Publishers.

1.3 Health equity audits

Health equity audits (HEAs) were first proposed in the 1998 Acheson Report:

> We RECOMMEND Directors of Public Health, working on behalf of health and local authorities, produce an equity profile for the population they serve, and undertake a triennial audit of progress towards achieving objectives to reduce inequalities in health. (Recommendation 39)

HEAs are therefore ongoing processes rather than static reviews; health equity profiles are simply the first stage of this audit process.

Public health authorities (largely within primary care trusts) have a duty to perform HEAs in order to understand, monitor and act on inequitable health circumstances within their areas and populations. It should be emphasised that these audits are regarding **inequity/equity** rather than **inequality/equality** (see **1.5** and **1.4** respectively). An HEA must therefore consider whether the distribution of a health outcome, risk factor or service is fair (equitable), not just whether it is consistent (equal) among different subgroups of the population. It should be noted that specific accounting rules for equity assessment are sometimes not explicit, in that the criteria for deciding if something represents an inequity are sometimes difficult to formulate and are often based on subjective principles. A study in East Anglia found the provision of surgery for non-small cell lung cancer to be inequitable because surgery was not provided according to the principle that provision should be proportionate to need (incidence) (Battersby et al, 2004). An HEA process could be used to address this mismatch between service need and provision, and to monitor whether action taken was effective in reducing that inequity.

References
Acheson, Sir Donald (1998) *Independent Inquiry into Inequalities in Health*, London: The Stationery Office (www.archive.official-documents.co.uk/document/doh/ih/ih.htm).
Battersby, J., Flowers, J. and Harvey, I. (2004) 'An alternative approach to quantifying and addressing inequity in healthcare provision: access to surgery for lung cancer in the east of England', *Journal of Epidemiology and Community Health*, vol 58, pp 623-5.

Further reading
Tudor Hart, J. (1971) 'The inverse care law', *The Lancet*, vol 1, pp 405-12.

Weblinks

Eastern Region Public Health Observatory HEA:
www.erpho.org.uk/topics/HEA

See also: 1.4 Inequality/equality; 1.5 Inequity/equity

1.4 Inequality/equality

Inequality is said to exist when there is a difference in the distribution of a resource (such as income) or outcome (such as mortality or educational achievement) across groups of people or places (for example, by socioeconomic group or by gender). For example, the rate of mortality from suicide may be higher for young men than for young women, or the rate of unemployment may be twice as high in one city as in another. It is thus a description of the differences between groups or areas. There is no consensus on what should be used to measure the extent of inequality. Any choice of inequality indicator involves implicit choices about which dimensions of inequality are important to capture (for an extended discussion see Harper and Lynch, 2006).

The term 'inequalities in health' can refer to a range of dimensions of inequality in health outcome – by gender, ethnicity, geography and so on. In the UK and Europe the term is most often used to refer to inequalities in health by socioeconomic position (SEP) while in the US it usually refers to differences in health among race/ethnic groups.

The term 'health variations' has sometimes been used in place of 'health inequalities'. Describing observed differences as 'variations' involves a rather more 'naturalistic' and dispassionate stance, focusing on description without judgement; 'inequalities' on the other hand are usually seen as something caused by modifiable differences in some exposure and so are something to be reduced.

Discussion point

I do not believe that one person's poverty is caused by another's wealth. (Michael Howard, then leader of the Conservative Party, in an advert in *The Independent*, 2 January 2004)

The poor of the world cannot be made rich by redistribution of wealth. Poverty can't be eliminated by punishing people who've escaped poverty, taking their money and giving it as a reward to people who have failed to escape. (P.J. O'Rourke, www.inequality.org/quotes.cfm)

All but the hard hearted man must be torn with pity for this pathetic dilemma of the rich man, who has to keep the poor man just stout enough to do the work and just thin enough to have to do it. (G.K. Chesterton, www.inequality.org/quotes.cfm)

References

Harper, S. and Lynch, J. (2006) *Methods for measuring cancer disparities: A review using data relevant to healthy people 2010 cancer-related objectives*, Washington DC: National Cancer Institute.

Further reading

Hills, J. and Stewart, K. (2005) *A more equal society? New Labour, inequality and exclusion*, Bristol: The Policy Press.

Hurrell, A. and Woods, N. (1999) *Inequality, globalization, and world politics*, Oxford: Oxford University Press.

Pantazis, C. and Gordon, D. (eds) (2000) *Tackling inequalities: Where are we now and what can be done?*, Bristol: The Policy Press.

Romero, M. and Margolis, E. (2005) *The Blackwell companion to social inequalities*, Oxford: Blackwell.

Wheeler, B., Shaw, M., Mitchell, R. and Dorling, D. (2005) *Life in Britain: Using millennial Census data to understand poverty, inequality and place*, Bristol: The Policy Press (www. shef.ac.uk/sasi/research/life_in_britain.htm). [A pack of 10 reports, a technical, summary and five posters produced for the Joseph Rowntree Foundation].

See also: 1.5 Inequity/equity

1.5 Inequity/equity

Inequity and equity refer to how *fairly* services, opportunities and access are distributed across groups of people or places, according to the need of that group. Inequities are said to occur when services do not reflect health needs.

For example, we could compare two groups of people, say manual and non-manual workers. If the need for hip replacements (indicated by severe and advanced arthritis) was such that the manual workers were twice as likely to need hip replacements than the non-manual workers, this would constitute an *inequality*. If the provision of hip replacements for manual workers reflected this need, with an operation rate for the manual workers at twice that of the non-manual workers, then *equity* would exist. However, if the rate of operations among the non-manual group is more than half that of the manual group, then *inequity* would exist as they would be more likely to be getting a hip replacement operation in response to their need than the manual group.

Equity is thus about providing services and distributing resources in response to, and in proportion to, need. Many health and other services, including the NHS, aim to pursue equity in the delivery of the services they provide.

Discussion point

'The world ... is not an inn, but a hospital,' said Sir Thomas Browne more than three and a half centuries ago, in 1643. That is a discouraging, if not entirely surprising, interpretation of the world from the distinguished author of *Religio Medici* and *Pseudodoxia Epidemia*. But Browne may not be entirely wrong: even today (not just in Browne's 17th-century England), illness of one kind or another is an important presence in the lives of a great many people. Indeed, Browne may have been somewhat optimistic in his invoking of a hospital: many of the people who are most ill in the world today get no treatment for their ailments, nor the use of effective means of prevention.

In any discussion of social equity and justice, illness and health must figure as a major concern. I take that as my point of departure – the ubiquity of health as a social consideration – and begin by noting that health equity cannot but be a central feature of the justice of social arrangements in general. The reach of health equity is immense. But there is a converse feature of this connection to which we must also pay attention. Health equity cannot be concerned only with health, seen in isolation. Rather it must come to grips with the larger issues of fairness and justice in social arrangements, including economic allocations, paying appropriate attention to the role of health in human life and freedom. Health equity is most certainly not just about the distribution of *health*, not to mention the even narrower focus on the distribution of *health care*. Indeed, health equity as a consideration has an enormously wide reach and relevance. (Sen, 2002, p 659)

References

Sen, A.K. (2002) 'Why health equity?', *Health Economics*, vol 11, no 8, pp 659-66.

Further reading

Anand, S., Peter, F. and Sen, A. (2004) *Public health, ethics, and equity*, Oxford: Oxford University Press.

Layer, G. (2005) *Closing the equity gap: The impact of widening participation strategies in the UK and the USA*, Leicester: National Institute of Adult Continuing Education.

Murray, A. and Davis, R. (2001) 'Equity in regional service provision', *Journal of Regional Science*, vol 41, no 4, pp 557-600.

Sassi, F., Le Grand, J. and Archard, L. (2001) 'Equity versus efficiency: a dilemma for the NHS', *BMJ*, vol 323, pp 762-3.

Shaw, M. and Dorling, D. (2004) 'Who cares in England and Wales? The positive care law: a cross-sectional study', *British Journal of General Practice*, vol 54, pp 899-903.

Wood, D., Clark, D. and Gatrell, A. (2004) 'Equity of access to adult hospice inpatient care within north-west England', *Palliative Medicine*, vol 18, no 6, pp 543-9.

See also: 1.4 Inequality/equality

1.6 Lay epidemiology

Lay epidemiology has been described as:

> ... [the process by which] ... individuals interpret health risks through the routine observation and discussion of cases of illness and death in personal networks and the public arena, as well as from formal and informal evidence arising from other sources, such as television and magazines. (Frankel et al, 1991, p 428)

The concept therefore refers to the conceptions held by members of the general public as opposed to epidemiological specialists. Lay epidemiology can refer to individuals' own understanding of patterns of health and illness and their causes, informed by anecdotal evidence, personal experience and interpretation of scientific and popular literature and media. Some researchers have used the term to refer to epidemiological studies carried out by, or in conjunction with, non-specialists, but the term 'popular epidemiology' is more generally used in these cases (see Example).

Strengths

An understanding of lay epidemiology can be crucial in order to convert scientific epidemiology into public health action that actually has an impact on the health of the population. For example, Lawlor et al (2003) suggest that appreciating processes of lay epidemiology may be the key to understanding the relatively limited impact of public health initiatives on smoking rates among populations of lower socioeconomic position (SEP) (compared with higher SEP groups). It is also a means by which communities or individuals that feel untrusting of health professionals and 'authorities', or disenchanted with health improvement processes, might have the opportunity to engage with organisations and processes that they otherwise would not.

Limitations

Lay epidemiology can sometimes be viewed as 'dumbed down' or 'unscientific', and discredited as such, by specialists or decision makers. This can often lead to a confrontational situation between scientists/authorities and communities or individuals that is not easy to rectify into a constructive relationship (see Weblinks).

Example

In the late 1990s, the Women's Environmental Network carried out a process and campaign called 'Putting Breast Cancer on the Map'. This involved asking women around the UK to draw maps indicating their interpretations of breast cancer rates and sources of environmental pollution that they considered may have some influence on those rates. While these kind of investigations do not necessarily fit within textbook definitions of epidemiological studies, their intent is not necessarily the same, and their importance in terms of how people understand and react to patterns of diseases can be great.

> ... the project ... received more than 300 maps. Women approached the task in a variety of creative ways, some drawing life maps to demonstrate exposure to pollutants in different places and stages of their lives, others drawing maps of their immediate home or work environment. The project identified a need in women to take part in positive action to bring about a change in the minds of government, the medical establishment, as well as society at large, in the way breast cancer is viewed, treated and politicised in the UK. (www.wen.org.uk/health/Mapping)

References
Frankel, S., Davison, C. and Davey Smith, G. (1991) 'Lay epidemiology and the rationality of responses to health education', *British Journal of General Practice*, vol 41, pp 428-30.
Lawlor, D.A., Frankel, S., Shaw, M., Ebrahim, S. and Davey Smith, G. (2003) 'Smoking and ill health: does lay epidemiology explain the failure of smoking cessation programs among deprived populations?', *American Journal of Public Health*, vol 93, no 2, pp 266-70.

Further reading
Allmark, P. and Tod, A. (2006) 'How should public health professionals engage with lay epidemiology?', *Journal of Medical Ethics*, vol 32, pp 460-3.
Watterson, A. (1994) 'Whither lay epidemiology in UK public health policy and practice? Some reflections on occupational and environmental health opportunities', *Journal of Public Health*, vol 16, no 3, pp 270-4.

Weblinks
For some views on the public understanding of science and relationships between specialists and non-specialists, see the following:
www.badscience.net
www.greenaudit.org

1.7 Life course socioeconomic position

Life course epidemiology is the study of the long-term biological, behavioural and psychosocial processes that link adult health and disease risk to physical or social exposures during gestation, childhood, adolescence, earlier in adult life or across generations (Ben Shlomo and Kuh, 2002).

Indicators of socioeconomic position (SEP) from different stages of the life course can be useful in examining how socioeconomic conditions operating at different stages of life may differentially influence disease risk. Some socioeconomic indicators are only valid at specific ages; for example, *education* is mostly completed by young adulthood, whereas *occupation* can only occur after the age of 16 in rich countries. However, the same indicator can be measured at different times during the life course: for example, father's *occupation* characterises childhood SEP, while first occupation, longest and last occupation can characterise early to later adulthood SEP. In other cases, an indicator may be more appropriate for a given period of time, as is the case of wealth, which may better characterise SEP at old age than occupation or other indicators. The following figure presents several indicators of SEP combined in a life course framework.

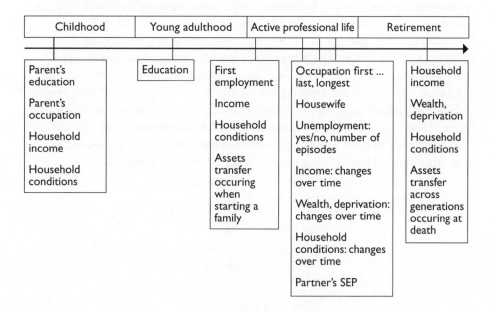

Uses of life course socioeconomic position

Since the meaning and therefore likely effect of socioeconomic conditions vary over time, having multiple measures of SEP over time can provide insight into the potential mechanisms that generate inequalities in health. For example, there is evidence that childhood SEP (often indexed by father's occupation) is particularly relevant in determining the risk of stomach cancer (Galobardes et al, 2004). This probably reflects the stage of the life course when the exposure causing this disease takes place – infection with the bacteria *H Pylori*, which occurs most commonly in childhood – and is associated with socioeconomic deprivation having an aetiological role in stomach cancer. By contrast there appears to be a cumulative effect of childhood and adulthood SEP on coronary heart disease (Galobardes et al, 2004).

Several models can be hypothesised to link life course exposures with adult disease (Ben Shlomo and Kuh, 2002). In the *critical period model*, of which the fetal programming hypothesis is an example (Barker and Robinson, 1993), an exposure acting at a specific time has long-lasting effects on the structure or function of the body. In contrast, the *accumulation of risk model* suggests that effects accumulate over the life course, and health damage increases with the duration and/or number of exposures. The latter model also allows for developmental *sensitive periods* during which susceptibility to future disease may be greater than at other time periods but that are not critical (that is, exposure at other time periods could also result in increased disease risk). The accumulation model seems to explain better how exposure to low SEP across different stages of the life course has additive effects in increasing disease risk (Davey Smith and Lynch, 2004). Accumulation of risk can also be due to clustering of exposures. For example, children from lower socioeconomic backgrounds are more likely to be of low birth weight, have poorer diets, be more exposed to passive smoking and some infectious agents, and have fewer educational opportunities (Ben Shlomo and Kuh, 2002). Finally, exposures may form *chains of risk*, where, for example, low educational attainment will increase the probability of a person working in an occupation with a high risk of toxic exposures and of having low income (Davey Smith and Lynch, 2004).

Difficulties in obtaining and interpreting associations with life course socioeconomic position

Measurement difficulties

The ideal life course study is one that has repeated measurements: from one's parents before conception, through gestation, childhood, early adulthood and then into late adulthood, when disease occurrence is most common. In reality there are very few such studies. While common health and disease outcomes are now increasingly available from some of the older birth cohorts, such as the British 1946 birth cohort (see www.nshd.mrc.ac.uk), other studies have relied on retrospective reporting of childhood social circumstances by adults many decades later. The accuracy of this information is unclear, but a study of individuals born in Aberdeen, Scotland, compared childhood social class collected at the time (based on father's occupation), with that retrospectively reported by the adults when they were in their late 40s/early 50s, and found only modest agreement between the two (Batty et al, 2005). The effect of misreporting varied by outcome, such that the associations of social class with birth weight and cognitive function were weaker when adult retrospective data were used rather than data collected at the time . However, the associations of childhood SEP with coronary heart disease and stroke were the same whichever method was used (Lawlor et al, 2006).

For individual SEP indicators, such as income, it would be desirable to have summary measures that indicated the entire income trajectory of an individual over time but these data are hard to obtain, and even if there are repeated measurements in a cohort they will inevitably cover only a certain portion of the life course each time. An extended array of life course indicators might include measures of parental SEP prior to birth and during childhood, own education, first job and then subsequent occupational history, income over time, asset accumulation and asset transfers from parents. Collecting such information then raises questions of how to create summary measures when each individual indicator is based on a different measurement scale as well as taken at different times and consequently in different contexts. The use of statistical techniques such as latent variable and structural equation modelling may be helpful in capturing these complicated processes (De Stavola et al, 2005).

Interpretation difficulties

There is an intrinsic problem in differentiating life course processes. Whether critical period, *social mobility*, accumulation of risks or combinations of these underlie the association between SEP and a health outcome requires prior knowledge of the specific causal mechanisms (Hallqvist et al, 2004). Comparing changes in the association or its magnitude with different socioeconomic indicators across the life course with the health outcome can point to certain exposures (as discussed above). But the interpretation of such findings can also be problematic. For example, a study based on census linkage in Norway among individuals who were aged 31-50 in 1990 compared the relative effects of childhood SEP, based on family and parental data from the 1960 census, to adult SEP based on similar data for the participant from the 1990 census (Claussen et al, 2003; Naess et al, 2004). All-cause and cause-specific mortality during a four-year follow-up period to 1994 were the outcomes. The difficulties here are that it is unclear whether any differences between the relative effects of childhood and adult SEP for different outcomes reflect different aetiological life course patterns or the different sources of bias inherent in the measurements at these two periods. In particular, the association of the childhood measurement would be influenced by survivor bias, since only those who survived to 1990 could possibly be included, whereas the 1990 measurement is influenced by reverse causality and downwards social mobility (particularly since the deaths were all within a period of four years following the adult measure). The impact of these different biases is likely to vary for different outcomes and may have in part explained some of the results.

References

Barker, D.J.P. and Robinson, R.J. (1993) *Fetal and infant origins of adult disease*, London: BMJ Books.

Batty, G.D., Lawlor, D.A., Macintyre, S., Clark, H. and Leon D.A. (2005) 'Accuracy of adults' recall of childhood occupational social class: evidence from the Aberdeen Children of the 1950s study', *Journal of Epidemiology and Community Health*, vol 59, pp 898-903.

Ben Shlomo, Y. and Kuh, D. (2002) 'A life course approach to chronic disease epidemiology: conceptual models, empirical challenges and interdisciplinary perspectives', *International Journal of Epidemiology*, vol 31, pp 285-93.

Claussen, B., Davey Smith, G. and Thelle, D. (2003) 'Impact of childhood and adulthood socioeconomic position on cause specific mortality: the Oslo Mortality Study', *Journal of Epidemiology and Community Health*, vol 57, pp 40-5.

Davey Smith, G. and Lynch, J. (2004) 'Life course approaches to socioeconomic differentials in health', in D. Kuh and Y. Ben-Shlomo, *A life course approach to chronic disease epidemiology* (2nd edn), Oxford: Oxford University Press.

De Stavola, B., Nitsch, D., dos Santos Silva, I., McCormack, V., Hardy, R., Mann, V., Cole, T.J., Morton, S. and Leon, D.A. (2005) 'Statistical issues in life course epidemiology', *American Journal of Epidemiology*, vol 163, pp 84-96.

Galobardes, B., Lynch, J.W. and Davey Smith, G. (2004) 'Childhood socioeconomic circumstances and cause-specific mortality in adulthood: systematic review and interpretation', *Epidemiologic Reviews*, vol 26, pp 7-21.

Hallqvist, J., Lynch, J., Bartley, M., Lang, T. and Blane, D. (2004) 'Can we disentangle life course processes of accumulation, critical period and social mobility? An analysis of disadvantaged socio-economic positions and myocardial infarction in the Stockholm Heart Epidemiology Program', *Social Science & Medicine*, vol 58, pp 1555-62.

Lawlor, D.A., Ronalds, G., Macintyre, S., Clark, H. and Leon, D.A. (2006) 'Family socioeconomic position at birth and future cardiovascular disease risk: findings from the Aberdeen Children of the 1950s Cohort Study', *American Journal of Public Health*, vol 96, pp 1271-7.

Naess, O., Claussen, B. and Davey Smith, G. (2004) 'Relative impact of childhood and adulthood socioeconomic conditions on cause specific mortality in men', *Journal of Epidemiology and Community Health*, vol 58, pp 597-8.

See also: 4.1 Age-period-cohort analysis (or effects)

1.8 Living standards

'Living standards' is a broad term encompassing the material conditions in which an individual, a community or a population lives. This comprises ownership of, or access to, goods, amenities and services, along with environmental circumstances such as housing conditions, and opportunities such as education or employment. These general living conditions are therefore wide-ranging, and may include luxuries, such as internet access, as well as those essential for life, such as nutrition and clean water. Living standards are often discussed in the context of income, wealth and poverty, often with an assumption that higher wealth and income are inevitably related to better living standards.

Discussion point

Official statistics show that average living standards are falling for the first time since Labour came to office in 1997.

The latest figures show prices up 3.7 percent, according to the RPI index, and earnings excluding bonuses up by only 3.5 percent. The last time the RPI exceeded earnings growth was in 1995, in the dying days of the Tories.

These dry numbers reflect what millions of workers feel in their bones – that the cost of everything is going through the roof and wages aren't keeping up. (*Socialist Worker*, 25 November 2006)

In the year to September [2006], pay growth (excluding bonuses) in the private sector was 3.6 per cent, compared with 3.2 per cent for the public sector. Including bonus payments, private sector growth stood at 4.0 per cent compared with 3.5 per cent for the public sector.

In the year to September 2006, consumer prices increased by 2.4 per cent, which is below the rate of earnings growth. (www.statistics.gov.uk)

Weblinks

The World Bank's Living Standards Measurement Study (primarily used in developing countries):
www.worldbank.org/lsms

See also: 1.10 Poverty; 1.20 Wealth; 2.16 Income

1.9 Official and vital statistics

Official statistics have been described as:

> ... statistics produced by government agencies to:
> * shed light on economic and social conditions
> * develop, implement and monitor policies
> * inform decision making, debate and discussion both within government and the wider community. (www.data-archive.ac.uk)

However, this definition varies, and is in some ways subjective. What is perceived as an 'official statistic' by one person or organisation may not be by another (see Statistics Commission, 2005). Vital statistics are a component of official statistics, and are perhaps more simply defined, although they may include different sets of information in different countries. They tend to be statistics related to 'vital' events, especially births, deaths and marriages. Other statistics that may be considered as 'vital' might include those on abortions, divorces, specific health events (such as stillbirths or cancer registrations) and population figures.

Many official and vital statistics are used in order to understand the socioeconomic circumstances of the population, and the relationships between these circumstances and health outcomes (see, for example, Drever and Whitehead, 1997).

Discussion point

The quality, potential for bias, and trustworthiness of official statistics is an ongoing debate in the UK. The Statistics Commission was set up in 2000 to 'help ensure that official statistics are trustworthy and responsive to public needs', to 'give independent, reliable and relevant advice' and by so doing to 'provide an additional safeguard on the quality and integrity' of official statistics (www.statscom.org.uk). However, in November 2006 the government published a Bill making the Office for National Statistics independent of government and run by a non-ministerial department, which takes on the role of the Statistics Commission.

Drawing on the findings from five discussion groups plus a review of decades of survey data, the MORI report shows that in this greater climate of distrust – driven by increased awareness of spin and the debates over the case for war with Iraq – public confidence in official statistics has diminished. The context for government information is also much more challenging than it used to be because of the huge growth in information available and an increasingly 'bitter and dismissive' media. (Ipsos MORI, 2005)

References

Drever, F. and Whitehead, M. (eds) (1997) *Decennial Supplement DS15: Health inequalities*, London: The Stationery Office.

Ipsos MORI (2005) *Who do you believe? Trust in government information* (www.ipsos-mori.com/trust/).

Statistics Commission (2005) *Report No 24: Official statistics: Perceptions and trust*, London: Statistics Commission (www.statscom.org.uk).

Further reading

Kerrison, S. and Macfarlane, A. (eds) (2000) *Official health statistics: An unofficial guide*, London: Arnold.

Weblinks

UK official and vital statistics:
England (and other countries):
  www.statistics.gov.uk
Northern Ireland:
  www.nisra.gov.uk/
Scotland:
  www.gro-scotlamd.gov.uk/
Wales:
  new.wales.gov.uk/topics/statistics/
Radical Statistics: www.radstats.org.uk

See also: 2.2 Benefit claimants; 2.23 National Statistics Socioeconomic Classification (NS-SEC); 2.28 Poverty – the official government measure; 3.4 Households Below Average Income (HBAI)

1.10 Poverty

There is no single definition of poverty. The term 'absolute poverty' is generally taken to refer to lack of basic resources required for daily living – food, water, clothing, shelter and so on. Alternatively, it may be defined as living below a certain income threshold (such as a dollar a day). In the context of developed (industrialised, rich) nations, when people refer to poverty they most often mean 'relative poverty', which is socially defined and very much dependent on context and cohort. Relative poverty occurs when the resources available to a person, household or area are so far below average levels that they are considered to be excluded from ordinary living patterns, customs and activities – that is, the term refers to whether people are poor in relation to the people around them. While absolute poverty focuses on access to essential material resources, the idea of relative poverty can additionally include access to other resources such as knowledge/education, and social and community participation.

Peter Townsend defined poverty as:

> ... the absence or inadequacy of those diets, amenities, standards, services and activities which are common or customary in society. (Townsend, 1979)

The European Union's working definition of poverty is:

> Persons, families and groups of persons whose resources (material, cultural and social) are so limited as to exclude them from the minimum acceptable way of life in the Member State to which they belong. (EEC, 1985)

Official measures of poverty, however, tend to focus on the measurement of relative income.

References
EEC (1985) 'On specific community action to combat poverty' (Council decision of 19 December 1984), 85/8/EEC, *Official Journal of the EEC*, 2/24.
Townsend, P. (1979) *Poverty in the United Kingdom*, London/Berkeley, CA: Allen Lane, Penguin/University of California Press.

Further reading
Spicker, P. (2007) *The idea of poverty*, Bristol: The Policy Press.

Weblinks

UK poverty statistics and resources:
www.poverty.org.uk
International perspectives:
www.worldbank.org/poverty

See also: 1.1 Deprivation; 1.15 Social exclusion; 1.20 Wealth; 2.7 Child poverty – the official government measure; 3.4 Households Below Average Income (HBAI)

1.11 Psychosocial factors

Psychosocial factors comprise a group of health risk factors, although this group contains some issues that may also be considered as outcomes, for example, stress or depression. These factors lie at the interface between the social and the psychological, and so imply a perceptual linkage between objective aspects of society and individual psychological reactions to those aspects of society. Martikainen and colleagues (2002) usefully distinguish macro, meso and micro levels. Macro-social structure includes ownership, legal, welfare and tax structures; meso-social formations include religious organisations, the family and clubs, while the micro level includes individual attributes. Psychosocial factors lie between the meso-level social formations and individual psychological characteristics. Commonly studied psychosocial factors include autonomy, control at work, social support, depression and social capital. There have also been efforts to measure perceptions of social rank. Psychosocial exposures are thought to affect health via two main pathways – by influencing health behaviours and by direct mechanisms involving psycho-neuro-endocrine-immune pathways.

Discussion point

To feel depressed, cheated, bitter, desperate, vulnerable, frightened, angry, worried about debts or job or housing insecurity; to feel devalued, useless, helpless, uncared for, hopeless, isolated, anxious and a failure: these feelings can dominate people's whole experience of life. (Wilkinson, 1996, p 215)

Social dominance, inequality, autonomy, and the quality of social relations have an impact on psychosocial wellbeing and are among the most powerful explanations for the pattern of population health in rich countries. (Marmot and Wilkinson, 2001, p 1233)

These results do not offer much support for a psychosocial environment theory as a general explanation for health differences between rich countries. Higher perceived control over life circumstances was actually substantially associated with higher CHD – the opposite of what would be predicted by the psychosocial environment theory and the opposite of what would be inferred from studies of individuals. (Lynch et al, 2001, p 199)

References

Martikainen, P., Bartley, M. and Lahelma, E. (2002) 'Psychosocial determinants of health in social epidemiology', *International Journal of Epidemiology*, vol 31, pp 1091-3.

Further reading

Hemingway, H., and Marmot, M. (1999) 'Evidence based cardiology: psychosocial factors in the aetiology and prognosis of coronary heart disease. Systematic review of prospective cohort studies', *BMJ*, vol 318, no 7196, pp 1460-7.

Kubzansky, L. and Kawachi, I. (2000) 'Going to the heart of the matter: do negative emotions cause coronary heart disease?', *Journal of Psychosomatic Research*, vol 48, no 4-5, pp 323-37.

Lynch, J., Davey Smith, G., Hillemeier, M., Shaw, M., Raghunathan, T. and Kaplan, G. (2001) 'Income inequality, the psychosocial environment, and health: comparisons of wealthy nations', *The Lancet*, vol 358, pp 194-200.

Macleod, J. and Davey Smith, G. (2003) 'Psychosocial factors and public health: a suitable case for treatment?', *Journal of Epidemiology and Community Health*, vol 57, no 8, pp 565-70.

Macleod, J., Davey Smith, G., Heslop, P., Metcalfe, C., Carroll, D. and Hart, C. (2001) 'Are the effects of psychosocial exposures attributable to confounding? Evidence from a prospective observational study on psychological stress and mortality', *Journal of Epidemiology and Community Health*, vol 55, no 12, pp 878-84.

Marmot, M. and Wilkinson, R. (2001) 'Psychosocial and material pathways in the relation between income and health: a response to Lynch et al', *BMJ*, vol 322, pp 1233-6.

Relman, A. and Angell, M. (2002) 'Resolved: psychosocial interventions can improve clinical outcomes in organic disease (Con)', *Psychosomatic Medicine*, vol 64, no 4, pp 558-63.

Wilkinson. R.G. (1996) *Unhealthy societies: The afflictions of inequality*, London: Routledge.

See also: 1.13 Social capital

1.12 Segregation

'Segregation' is another term for 'separation', and it is used in the context of socioeconomic inequalities to describe the geographical separation between communities or populations of different socioeconomic position (SEP); most frequently it is used in the US to refer to racial or ethnic residential segregation. Throughout recent British history, households and people of similar SEP have tended to be spatially concentrated (see, for example, Rowntree, 1901); people are more likely to live near to people similar to themselves than to people very different from themselves. The processes that result in this social segregation are not simply based on choices made by individuals, but also involve factors acting at local and national levels. These include housing and labour markets, planning policies and more general social policy (Meen et al, 2005).

At the macro level, the British North–South divide is a conspicuous example of geographical segregation; the North tends to be more deprived and have worse health than the South (Townsend et al, 1988; Shaw et al, 1999). However, segregation can operate at a variety of scales, and even within relatively affluent areas of Britain there exist concentrated pockets of relative poverty (Dorling et al, 2007).

Example

Research using the 2001 Census has demonstrated the geographical segregation of households with regard to their access to a car, an important measure of SEP (see **2.5 Car ownership and access**). Households that might need a car, but do not have one, were defined as those with dependent children, but without access to or ownership of a car. Households that may have more cars than they actually need were defined as those with three or more cars (one fifth of these households consisted of one or two people; two thirds had two or fewer employed people). The graph shows that these two groups, each of which contains around a million households, tend to live in different areas. The **Dissimilarity Index** (see **3.2**) for households that might need a car is 0.22, meaning that 22% of these households would need to be geographically redistributed to other areas in order to produce an even distribution across the UK. The equivalent Dissimilarity Index for households that might have more cars than needed is similar, at 0.18 (18%).

Households that might need a car, versus those that might have more cars than they need (2001 Census, UK)

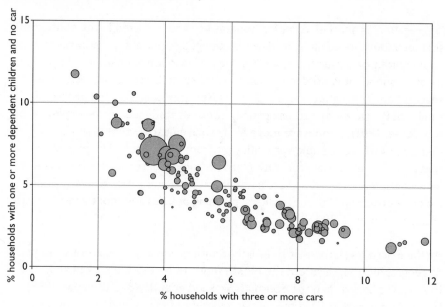

Note: Rates are calculated for 142 counties, unitary authorities and former metropolitan authorities and Northern Ireland (circle areas are proportional to population).
Source: Wheeler et al (2005)

Segregation may also be non-spatial; people of different SEP may live and work close to each other, but social structures may result in them not mixing in any meaningful way. 'Segregation' can also be used to refer to the unequal distribution of some characteristic or experience across different groups; people within different social classes could be thought of as 'segregated' by their differing experiences of poor health.

Measures often used to give an indication of the extent of segregation are the **Dissimilarity Index** (see **3.2**) and the **Gini coefficient** (see **3.3**). The alternative to segregation is 'integration', implying greater mixing of different groups in terms of geography and/or experience.

Discussion point: The North–South divide

Thousands of deaths from cancer might be prevented each year by reducing the north–south divide in terms of poverty, smoking and drinking, experts said yesterday.... Coincidentally, the British Heart Foundation published statistics yesterday suggesting similar north–south divides in heart disease. For example, the death rates for men and women under 75 were 67% and 84% higher in Scotland than in south-west England. (Meikle, 2005)

We expect GDP growth in the UK to accelerate and extend its gap over the western European average. We also expect the north–south divide to deepen further, with the gap between the best-performing and worst-performing UK regions more extreme than in any other western European country. We are seeing the continuation of a two-speed Britain with half of the 10 fastest-growing European regions over the next five years belonging to the UK. By contrast, some of the slowest growing European regions are also likely to be in the UK. (Economist Rebecca Snow, quoted in Willis, 2004)

References

Dorling, D., Rigby, J., Wheeler, B., Ballas, D., Thomas, B., Fahmy, E., Gordon, D. and Lupton, R. (2007) *Poverty, wealth and place in Britain 1968 to 2005: Understanding the transformation of the prospects of places*, York: Joseph Rowntree Foundation.

Meen, G., Gibb, K., Goody, J., McGrath, T. and Mackinnon, J. (2005) *Economic segregation in England: Causes, consequences and policy*, Bristol: The Policy Press.

Meikle, J. (2005) 'Cancer atlas reveals north-south divide', *The Guardian*, 6 July.

Rowntree, B.S. (1901) *Poverty: A study of town life*, Centennial edition published 2001, Bristol: The Policy Press.

Shaw, M., Dorling, D., Gordon, D. and Davey Smith, G. (1999) *The widening gap: Health inequalities and policy in Britain*, Bristol: The Policy Press.

Townsend, P., Phillimore, P. and Beattie, A. (1988) *Health and deprivation: Inequality and the North*, London: Croom Helm.

Wheeler, B., Shaw, M., Mitchell, R. and Dorling, D. (2005) *Life in Britain: Using millennial Census data to understand poverty, inequality and place*, Bristol: The Policy Press (www.shef.ac.uk/sasi/research/life_in-britain.htm) [A pack of 10 reports, a technical summary and five posters produced for the Joseph Rowntree Foundation].

Willis, B. (2004) 'North-south divide set to widen', *The Guardian*, 13 August.

Further reading

Duncan, O. and Duncan, B. (1955) 'A methodological analysis of segregation indices', *American Sociological Review*, vol 20, pp 210-17.

See also: 3.2 Dissimilarity Index; 3.3 Gini coefficient; 3.6 Measures of average disproportionality

1.13 Social capital

Social capital is one of the most prominently studied psychosocial factors (see 1.11). While there is no agreed definition of social capital, current conceptualisations encompass the ideas of bonding, bridging and linking social capital. Bonding social capital, most notably associated with the work of Robert Putnam, is the most restricted conceptualisation based on the extent of social networks and associated norms of reciprocity among individuals that helps generate shared identity. Bridging social capital involves networks that connect individuals who do not necessarily share an identity but involve social connections that foster mutual trust and generate social goods. Linking social capital is a special case of bridging social capital and refers to the sorts of social connections that run across formal or institutional power imbalances. Moving from bonding to bridging to linking social capital implies a move from more horizontal social relations among friends and family, to more vertical social relations that may cut across class, race/ethnic and gender groups where there are inherent differences in power, access to and control of resources. In public health, social capital is usually considered to be the property of a group rather than individuals.

Discussion point

We have always said that human capital is at the core of the new economy. But increasingly it is also social capital that matters too – the capacity to get things done, to cooperate, the magic ingredient that makes all the difference.

Too often in the past government programmes damaged social capital – sending in the experts but ignoring community organisations, investing in bricks and mortar but not in people. In the future we need to invest in social capital as surely as we invest in skills and buildings. (Tony Blair, Keynote speech, NCVO conference, 1999)

Among the competing discourses of social exclusion that emerged in the 1990s, the notion of social capital has taken hold and entered the vocabulary of national and local politics, and is now frequently invoked as a resource to be harnessed and promoted. In the UK, this popularity stems initially from the use of the term by Tony Blair in 1995 and later (King and Wickham-Jones, 1999), and wider adoption has followed the Social Exclusion Unit's references to social capital in their influential reports (SEU, 1998, 1999). While the term is gaining currency, it remains poorly understood…. Given the enthusiasm for social capital that local government is currently expressing in the UK, the need for more effective measures of the theoretical construct seems highly apposite. With few exceptions, existing approaches to the measurement of social capital hold little efficacy for political interpretations. (Roberts and Roche, 2001)

References

Roberts, M. and Roche, M. (2001) 'Quantifying social capital: measuring the intangible in the local policy context', *Radical Statistics*, vol 76, pp 15-28.

Further reading

Kawachi, I. and Berkman, L. (2000) 'Social cohesion, social capital, and health', in L.F. Berkman and I. Kawachi (eds) *Social epidemiology*, New York, NY: Oxford University Press, pp 174-90.

Kawachi, I., Kennedy, B., Lochner, K. and Prothrow-Stith, D. (1997) 'Social capital, income inequality, and mortality', *American Journal of Public Health*, vol 87, pp 1491-9.

King, D. and Wickham-Jones, M. (1999) 'Social capital, British social democracy and New Labour', *Democratization*, vol 6, pp 181-213.

Pearce, N. and Davey Smith, G. (2003) 'Is social capital the key to inequalities in health?', *American Journal of Public Health*, vol 93, pp 122-9.

Putnam, R. (2000) *Bowling Alone: America's declining social capital*, New York, NY: Simon & Schuster.

Sampson, R., Raudenbush, S. and Earls, F. (1997) 'Neighborhoods and violent crime: a multilevel study of collective efficacy', *Science*, vol 277, pp 918-24.

SEU (Social Exclusion Unit) (1998) *Bringing Britain together: A national strategy for neighbourhood renewal*, Cm 4045, London: The Stationery Office.

SEU (1999) *Annual Report*, Cm 4342, London: The Stationery Office.

Szreter, S. and Woolcock, M. (2004) 'Health by association? Social capital, social theory, and the political economy of public health', *International Journal of Epidemiology*, vol 33, pp 650-67.

See also: 1.11 Psychosocial factors

1.14 Social class

A variety of conceptualisations of social class exist. The key theoretical background for the concept of social class is the ideas of Karl Marx, where society is seen as divided according to those who do and those who do not own the means of production. Marx defined the 'working class', or proletariat, as members of society who sell their labour for wages, but do not own the means of production.

In practice, in the UK and elsewhere, 'social class' is frequently used more loosely (in a theoretical sense) and interchangeably with terms such as 'socioeconomic position' (SEP) and 'socioeconomic status' in the epidemiological literature. The British Registrar General's occupational classification (see **2.26**) is usually referred to as 'Social Classes', dividing the working population into six categories according to occupation, from 'professional' (such as lawyers and doctors) to 'unskilled manual' (such as builder's labourers).

Discussion point

The proportion of people who say they are middle-class has risen by nearly half in 40 years, a report says.

Forty-three percent of people surveyed said they were middle-class, compared with 30% of people in 1966.

But most – 53% – said they were working-class. The report also suggests that many are confused about which class they belong to ... the survey found that 36% of builders questioned regarded themselves as being middle-class, while 29% of bank managers said they were working-class. (BBC, 2006)

References
BBC (2006) 'More claiming middle-class status' (http://news.bbc.co.uk), 5 May.

Further reading
Engels, F. (1987) *The condition of the working class in England*, Harmondsworth: Penguin Books (originally published 1845).

Marx, K. (1993) *Capital: Critique of political economy. Vols 1, 2 and 3*, Harmondsworth: Penguin Books (originally published in 1867).

Veblen, T. (1994) *The theory of the leisure class*, London: Penguin Books (originally published 1899).

Wright, E.O. (1997) *Class counts: Comparative studies in class analysis*, Cambridge: Cambridge University Press.

1.15 Social exclusion

'Social exclusion' is a term that emerged in the 1990s as an additional, perhaps alternative, term to 'poverty' and 'deprivation'. There is no single agreed definition of social exclusion. Room and colleagues have described it as:

> ... multidimensional disadvantage which is of substantial duration and which involves dissociation from the major social and occupational milieux of society. (Room et al, 1993, p 72)

The UK government's definition is as follows:

> Social exclusion is about more than income poverty. Social exclusion happens when people or places suffer from a series of problems such as unemployment, discrimination, poor skills, low incomes, poor housing, high crime, ill health and family breakdown. When such problems combine they can create a vicious cycle. Social exclusion can happen as a result of problems that face one person in their life. But it can also start from birth. Being born into poverty or to parents with low skills still has a major influence on future life chances. (www.socialexclusion.gov.uk, 21 November 2006)

It is generally agreed that social exclusion is multidimensional and that it encompasses themes of participation in mainstream society and the realisation of social rights. Percy-Smith (2000) has outlined seven dimensions of social exclusion:

- economic (such as long-term unemployment; workless households; income poverty)
- social (such as homelessness; crime; disaffected youth)
- political (such as disempowerment; lack of political rights; alienation from/ lack of confidence in political processes)
- neighbourhood (such as decaying housing stock; environmental degradation)
- individual (such as mental and physical ill health; educational under-achievement)
- spatial (such as concentration/marginalisation of vulnerable groups)
- group (concentration of above characteristics in particular groups, such as disabled, elderly, minority ethnic).

The term 'social inclusion' is used to capture the strategies employed to counter the processes and effects of social exclusion and to achieve a more inclusive society; more specifically it is used to refer to reducing the inequalities gap between the least advantaged groups and communities and the rest of society by closing the opportunity gap and ensuring that support reaches those that need it most.

References

Percy-Smith, J. (ed) (2000) *Policy responses to social exclusion: Towards inclusion?*, Buckingham: Open University Press.

Room, G. et al (1993) *Anti-poverty action-research in Europe*, Bristol: School for Advanced Urban Studies, University of Bristol.

Further reading

Hills, J. and Stewart, K. (eds) (2005) *A more equal society? New Labour, poverty, inequality and exclusion*, Bristol: The Policy Press.

Pantazis, C., Gordon, D. and Levitas, R. (eds) (2005) *Poverty and social exclusion in Britain: The Millennium Survey*, Bristol: The Policy Press.

Ridge, T. (2002) *Childhood poverty and social exclusion: From a child's perspective*, Bristol: The Policy Press.

Weblinks

The government's Social Exclusion Unit, part of the Cabinet Office: www.socialexclusion.gov.uk/

CASE, the ESRC Research Centre for the Analysis of Social Exclusion: http://sticerd.lse.ac.uk/case/

Supported by the New Policy Institute and the Joseph Rowntree Foundation, this site contains statistics on poverty and social exclusion: www.poverty.org.uk/

See also: 1.1 Deprivation; 1.10 Poverty

1.16 Social mobility

Social mobility describes the movement (or opportunities for movement) of groups and individuals between different social groups. The extent or range of social mobility varies in different societies. Feudal and caste societies are generally considered to be closed societies in which there is little opportunity for individual mobility (although group mobility may occur; see Examples). An individual's position in these societies was largely based on ascribed characteristics (family origin, gender, ethnic group). These ascribed characteristics are still socially significant in modern societies, but modern Britain tends to place greater emphasis on achievement and as a result is more open to individual social mobility.

A society that is considered to be open and supportive of mobility is often considered to have advantages over socially rigid societies. These advantages relate to several domains:

Association with health improvement: although *life course* studies suggest an enduring effect of one's social origins, it is also true that individuals who move up the social stratum (through either *intergenerational* or *intragenerational* mobility; see Examples) have better health outcomes (Lawlor et al, 2002) although the converse is also the case.

Equality of opportunity: the ability of individuals or groups to move through (in particular up) the social stratum implies equality of opportunity.

Economic efficiency: a society that supports social mobility is more likely to make best use of everyone's knowledge and skills than one that does not.

Social inclusion: social inclusion may be improved if individuals have the opportunity to move between social groups, although large amounts of movement may be detrimental to cohesion and inclusion.

However, it is also the case that societies with a large amount of individual mobility in income (especially over short periods of time) can result in economic instability and its associated social tensions. Furthermore, societies characterised by a high level of social mobility with the highest rewards going to those with greatest merit (however described) could result in large inequalities and socially marginalised groups.

Examples

Social mobility has been subclassified or used in a number of ways:

1. Group or individual mobility
The movement of a whole group up or down the social stratum usually occurs as a result of technological advance and/or large changes to the main political, religious or cultural influences in a society. Historical evidence of the Indian caste system suggests that the Brahmins did not always hold the position of indisputable superiority that they have held during the last two thousand years (Sorokin, 1959). Prior to this period, the caste of the warriors and rulers (the Kshatriyas) were superior. The elevation of the rank of the Brahmin caste as a whole through the ranks of other castes is an example of group social ascent.

Similarly, before the recognition of the Christian religion by Constantine the Great, the position of the Christian clergy was not a high one among other social ranks of Roman society (Sorokin, 1959). In the next few centuries the Christian Church, as a whole, experienced an enormous elevation of social position and rank. As a result of this wholesale elevation of the Christian Church, members of the clergy, and especially the high Church dignitaries, were elevated to the highest ranks of medieval society. By contrast the decrease in the authority of the Christian Church during recent times in the UK has led to a relative social decline for the group of Christian clergy.

Individual mobility is influenced by education, learning of specific skills and knowledge, marriage and broader social influences. Individual mobility can be within one's lifetime or in comparison to one's family origins (see below).

2. Horizontal (movement between social groups of same status) or vertical (movement to groups of different status) mobility
In its broadest sense social mobility refers to movement between any social group; hence movement between different religious or citizen groups would be examples of horizontal movement, as would movement from one job to another that did not represent a change in social or economic status. Vertical movement by contrast implies movement between social groups of different status. This can be divided into *ascending mobility* (also known as *upwards social mobility* or *social climbing*)

or descending mobility (also known as *downwards social mobility* or *social sinking*).

3. Intergenerational (children compared with parents) or intragenerational (within one's own lifetime) mobility
In Britain and most other industrialised countries there has been considerable absolute upwards intergenerational mobility, with subsequent generations being in higher income and social groups compared with previous generations. For example, in the British Women's Heart and Health Study (Lawlor et al, 2002), a cohort study of over 4,000 women aged 60-79 years in 2000, over 75% of the women's fathers were in manual occupational social classes whereas under 50% of their husbands were.

In open societies there is potential for many changes in social position across one's lifetime (intragenerational mobility) and few studies have detailed repeated measurements of socioeconomic position (SEP) across an individual's lifetime. In a prospective cohort study of Scottish working men, information was available on inter- and intragenerational mobility (Davey Smith et al, 1997). The majority (59%) of these men remained in the same social class at two time points in their adult life, with this also being the same as their father's social class. Forty-two per cent had fathers in manual social classes, and they themselves were in manual social classes at the time of their first job and in middle age (17% had non-manual for all three measurements). Sixteen per cent of men moved from manual to non-manual social classes in their adult life, while 5% moved from non-manual to manual. Further, the study found that SEP over the lifetime affected health and risk of premature death, but the relative importance of influences at different life stages and of different patterns of mobility varied for different health outcomes and causes of death.

4. Sociological literature tends to define social mobility in terms of movements between social classes or occupational groups, while the economic literature tends to define social mobility in terms of movements between income groups
Income has an advantage as a direct measure of command over resources but social class and occupation may be better measurements of life chances. It is important to note that mobility between income groups does not necessarily result in concomitant mobility between social class or occupational groups (and vice versa). For example, one's salary can increase with no associated increase in social status.

References

Davey Smith, G., Hart, C., Blane, D., Gillis, C. and Hawthorne V. (1997) 'Lifetime socioeconomic position and mortality: prospective observational study', *BMJ*, vol 314, pp 547-52.

Lawlor, D.A., Ebrahim, S. and Davey Smith G. (2002) 'Socioeconomic position in childhood and adulthood and insulin resistance: cross sectional survey using data from the British Women's Heart and Health Study', *BMJ*, vol 325, pp 805-7.

Sorokin, P. (1959) *Social and cultural mobility*, New York, NY: The Free Press.

Further reading

Heath, A. and Payne, C. (2000) 'Social mobility', in A.H. Halsey and J. Webb (eds) *Twentieth century British social trends*, Basingstoke, Macmillan, pp 254-78.

See also: 1.7 Life course socioeconomic position; 1.14 Social class; 1.17 Social status; 2.25 Occupation-based measures

1.17 Social status

'Social status' is used to indicate the 'social standing' or the prestige attached to one's position or role in society. The main source of social status in contemporary British society is arguably the work that someone does. Thus, an individual's social status can be measured with, or at least indicated by, an occupational-based indicator that groups occupations together based on the degree of prestige they are deemed to hold in society. The Registrar General's Occupational Social Classes schema is commonly used to infer social status in the UK, although in theoretical terms class and status are considered to be distinct. In common usage the term 'social status' is generally used to refer to a person's position in the social structure – and the importance that others ascribe to them. This closely corresponds to the degree to which an individual has power, influence, or a position of leadership in his or her social group.

Further reading
Marmot, M. (2004) *Status syndrome: How your social standing directly affects your health*, London: Bloomsbury.
Wilkinson, R.G. (1996) *Unhealthy societies: The afflictions of inequality*, London: Routledge.

See also: 1.14 Social class; 1.18 Social stratification; 2.25 Occupation-based measures

1.18 Social stratification

Social stratification refers to the hierarchically organised structures of social inequality that can be observed between groups of people in a society. Social stratification and inequality are inextricably linked, in that any system of stratification will, by definition, involve some social inequality between groups (note that this is different from the idea that a particular form or level of inequality is inevitable). Stratification can be used to distinguish various forms of social ranking or status groups, such as social class, gender and ethnicity. It is a particularly useful term when referring to contrasting systems of stratification in different settings or at different times. When considering forms of stratification we can focus on the things that members of a group have in common (see, for example, **1.13 Social capital**; **2.4 Cambridge Social Interaction and Stratification Scale (CAMSIS)**) or things that distinguish them (see, for example, **1.14 Social class**; **1.15 Social exclusion**).

See also: 1.4 Inequality/equality; 1.17 Social status

1.19 Status inconsistency

'Status inconsistency' refers to a situation where two assessments of status are at different levels leading to an atypical combination of status characteristics. The general concept has, within health studies, particularly been related to differences between education and later occupational social position, when it is referred to as 'status incongruity', or to different socioeconomic characteristics of spouses, when it is referred to as 'status discrepancy' (Kasl and Cobb, 1969; Vernon and Buffler, 1988). With respect to status incongruity a series of studies, largely carried out in the 1960s, considered that people who had, for example, higher levels of education than necessary for their occupational level, would experience psychosocial consequences that would be detrimental to their health. An alternative interpretation of effects of differences between childhood social circumstances and adulthood social circumstances was advanced by Forsdahl (1977) when he postulated that people who grew up in economically deprived circumstances would be more susceptible to factors like a high calorie diet when living as adults in relatively favourable social circumstances.

There has been rather less research on the psychosocial aspects of status inconsistency in more recent decades, possibly because no robust findings demonstrating particular adverse consequences of such inconsistency emerged (Vernon and Buffler, 1988). The Forsdahl hypothesis, however, stimulated a large body of research, starting with the replication of Forsdahl's original finding by David Barker and Clive Osmond in 1986, in the first paper in an influential series of studies on what became known as the Barker 'fetal origins' or 'developmental origins' of adult disease hypothesis. This suggested that very early life, including antenatal factors, influenced later health. However, in many post-Forsdahl formulations of this hypothesis the interaction between early life circumstances and any later life circumstances was relatively downplayed and the main effect of deprivation-related exposures in early life became key.

References

Barker, D. and Osmond C. (1986) 'Infant mortality, childhood nutrition and ischaemic heart disease in England and Wales', The Lancet, vol 1, pp 1077-81.

Forsdahl, A. (1977) 'Are poor living conditions in childhood and adolescence an important risk factor for atherosclerotic heart disease?', British Journal of Preventive Medicine, vol 31, pp 91-5.

Kasl, S. and Cobb, S. (1969) 'The intrafamilial transmission of rheumatoid arthritis. VI. Association of rheumatoid arthritis with several types of status inconsistency', *Journal of Chronic Diseases*, vol 22, pp 259-78.

Vernon, S. and Buffler, P. (1988) 'The status of status inconsistency', *Epidemiologic Reviews*, vol 10, pp 65-86.

See also: 1.7 Life course socioeconomic position; 1.16 Social mobility; 1.17 Social status

1.20 Wealth

Wealth is a measure of the total value of the accumulated assets owned by an individual, household, community or country. At the individual level, it combines assets and income that are accumulated throughout a person's life. In addition to income, wealth includes financial and physical assets such as the value of housing, cars, investments, inheritance or pension rights. The relative importance of wealth compared to income alone changes over the life course (wealth being more important in older age due to the accumulation of wealth and the impact of retirement on income), and is different for population subgroups – groups may have similar levels of income but very different levels of wealth.

It is very unusual for studies of health and inequality to measure wealth directly and, arguably, impossible to measure it completely; this is why we have labelled this a 'key concept' related to socioeconomic position (SEP) rather than a 'measure' of SEP, as that is how it is usually used. Some work that has measured wealth inequality has found similar patterns to those measuring inequality from a poverty/deprivation perspective. For example, a study of wealth in Britain between 1991 and 2001 found that the wealthiest 10% of the population experienced an increase in their holdings from 47% to 56% of national wealth over this decade (IPPR, 2004). The wealthy have also been theorised in a similar manner to 'the poor'; while the poor can be thought of as those who, through lack of resources, are excluded from contemporary societal norms, the wealthy can be thought of as those with sufficient resources to exclude themselves from societal norms (such as state education and health services, standard-class travel and so on) (Scott, 1994). This definition, complementary to that used to define poverty, enables theoretically robust measures of wealth to be developed (Dorling et al, 2007).

Discussion point

Discussions about health inequalities and inequities are most commonly concerned with poverty and its impact on health. The gaze of public health researchers is firmly on who lives in poverty, where, and for how long. The wealthy escape this detailed scrutiny and very rarely feature in causal explanations about why health inequities persist or in policy prescriptions to do something to redress inequities. At a time when the distribution of wealth is growing ever more unequal wealth should become a concern of epidemiologists, health political economists, and social policy makers. (Baum, 2005, p 542)

References

Baum, F. (2005) 'Wealth and health: the need for more strategic public health research', *Journal of Epidemiology and Community Health*, vol 59, pp 542-5.

Dorling, D., Rigby, J., Wheeler, B., Ballas, D., Thomas, B., Fahmy, E., Gordon, D. and Lupton, R. (2007) *Poverty, wealth and place in Britain 1968 to 2005: Understanding the transformation of the prospects of places*, York: Joseph Rowntree Foundation.

IPPR (Institute for Public Policy Research) (2004) 'Fairer inheritance tax needed to respond to rising wealth inequality', 22 August (www.ippr.org.uk/pressreleases/archive.asp?id=812), 24 November 2006.

Scott, J. (1994) *Poverty and wealth: Citizenship, deprivation and privilege*, London: Longman.

Further reading

Dorling, D., Shaw, M. and Davey Smith, G. (2006) 'Global inequalities and life expectancy due to AIDS', *BMJ*, vol 332, pp 662-4.

Kawachi, I. and Howden Chapman, P. (2004) 'Five American authors on wealth, poverty and inequality', *Journal of Epidemiology and Community Health*, vol 58, pp 738-42.

Lansley, S. (2006) *Rich Britain: The rise and rise of the new super-wealthy*, London: Politico's Publishing Ltd.

Veblen, T. (1994) *The theory of the leisure class*, London: Penguin Books (originally published 1899).

See also: 1.10 Poverty; 2.15 Housing wealth; 2.16 Income

Part Two
Measures of socioeconomic position

2.1 Amenities

A number of household amenities (or assets) are used as markers of material circumstances. These often include features such as access to hot and cold water in the house, having central heating and carpets, sole use of bathrooms and toilets, whether the toilet is inside or outside the home, and having a refrigerator, washing machine, or telephone. These household amenities are seen as direct measures of socioeconomic position (SEP) but they may also be seen as important because they may be associated with health outcomes through specific aetiological mechanisms. For example, lack of running water or lack of a household toilet may be associated with increased risk of infection.

The meaning of these amenities will vary by context and cohort. Very few people in contemporary advanced industrial societies will be without running hot water, an indoor toilet or bathroom facilities and, therefore, these measures are not able to differentiate individuals within these populations. However, such measures may still have relevance as indicators of childhood SEP among older adults living in the UK.

The census in the UK has traditionally included questions on household amenities. In 1971, for example, it included whether the household had a cooker, sink, bath/shower, toilet and central heating. The list of amenities included has decreased since 1971, reflecting the fact that some amenities have become features of virtually all households and hence no longer distinguish SEP.

Type of amenities included in last four UK censuses

Amenity	1971	1981	1991	2001
Car	•	•	•	•
Cooker	•			
Sink	•			
Bath/shower	•	•	•	Combined
Toilet	•	•	•	
Central heating			•	•

In non-industrialised countries, assets that have been used as indicators of SEP in health-related research include the number of livestock, owning a bicycle, refrigerator, radio, sewing machine, television or clock. For example, a study in Jaffna, Sri Lanka, measured the following amenities (Elankumuran et al, 2000):

1. Value of furniture available
2. Value of electrical items available
3. Value of equipment available
4. Value of vehicles available

They reported great variations in values suggesting that household amenities along with housing facilities could be a socioeconomic factor able to discriminate between families.

Strengths

Asking people about their household amenities is relatively straightforward (compared to the far more complicated coding of occupations, for example) and is less sensitive than asking about income or wealth. The inclusion of certain amenities in the census means that it is available in resources such as the ONS Longitudinal Study, which has great potential for epidemiological application (see weblink below).

Limitations

Measures of household amenities are not available for certain groups, such as those in communal establishments. There can also be problems in interpretation and the assumption that a household amenity is equally accessible to all household members. For instance, it may be problematic using household measures for older people who have moved in with their adult children, because the household circumstances are more a reflection of the child's social position than their own.

References

Elankumaran, C., Nithiyanandam, V., Ganesalingam, S. and Ganesh, S. (2000) 'New dimensions of parameters of poverty: an analysis of the Jaffna socioeconomic health study 1999 in Sri Lanka', International Development Studies Network (DEVNET) Conference on Poverty, Prosperity and Progress, Victoria University of Wellington, New Zealand, 17-19 November (www.devnet.org.nz).

Further reading

Howden-Chapman, P. (2004) 'Housing standards: a glossary of housing and health', *Journal of Epidemiology and Community Health*, vol 58, pp 162-8.

Shaw, M. (2004) 'Housing and public health', *Annual Review of Public Health*, vol 25, pp 397-418.

Weblinks

Office for National Statistics Longitudinal Study:
www.celsius.lshtm.ac.uk

Census:
www.statistics.gov.uk/census

See also: 2.5 Car ownership and access; 2.12 Housing conditions

2.2 Benefit claimants

The proportion of a population claiming or entitled to certain benefits, or whose income is derived solely from benefits, can be used as indicators of low income and lack of material resources (and therefore low socioeconomic position [SEP] and likely poverty). Each country will have its own particular package of benefits. These benefits can be used on their own or as components in indices of deprivation and are most often used to describe and compare areas. For example, in the UK, some of the benefits that are commonly used for this purpose are:

- *Income Support:* this is a benefit that can be claimed by people aged under 60 (people aged 60 or over can claim the Minimum Income Guarantee) who are on a low income and either not working or working less than 16 hours a week.
- *Income-based Jobseeker's Allowance (unemployment benefit):* this is paid to those capable of working, available for work and actively seeking work.
- *Housing Benefit and Council Tax Benefit:* Housing Benefit is a means-tested benefit payable to people on low incomes who are in rented accommodation (it excludes owner-occupiers). Council Tax Benefit is a means-tested benefit payable to any household (tenant or owner-occupier) below a defined level of income.
- *Free school meals:* these are available to school-age children in families whose parents or guardians receive Income Support.
- *In receipt of tax credits:* there are a range of tax credits that could be used, for example, Working Families Tax Credit, Child Tax Credit, Disabled Person's Tax Credit. Some are useful for identifying particular groups of people in need (for example, disabled people) whereas others, such as the Working Families Tax Credit, taper and can be paid to people with a relatively high level of income, and are thus not necessarily a good indicator of poverty or low SEP.

Often the proportion of claimants in particular vulnerable groups, such as pensioner households or households with dependent children, are calculated. Child Benefit is a 'universal benefit' paid to all children and thus cannot be used to discriminate between poorer and better-off households with children.

Strengths

The main advantage of such measures is that robust data are available for these means-tested benefits and they are frequently updated – the Department for Work and Pensions releases quarterly summary statistics on these and other benefits.

Limitations

Measures based on benefit claimants only tell us about one end of the socioeconomic spectrum. In addition, only those who actually claim the benefits, not all those who are eligible, are included. Due to the stigma that may be attached to various benefits (such as free school meals) some people may not claim everything to which they are entitled. Any changes to the benefit system and who is eligible to claim, over time, make it difficult to track trends; such changes tend to be frequent. Moreover, the number and proportion of people claiming benefits simply reflects the current rules as defined by the government – they are thus somewhat arbitrary indicators of low income, not defined by any scientific definition of what constitutes 'poverty'. A study by Morris et al (2000) estimated the minimum income necessary for 'healthy living' for a single, healthy man aged 18-30 and found that social security benefits at the time were less than half of that minimum. Similar work has focused on older people (Morris et al, 2005) and similarly found the minimum income for healthy living for older people to be higher than the pension credit guarantee.

Discussion point

On unemployment statistics ...

It is well known that the claimant count is misleadingly low. It includes only people entitled to unemployment-related benefits; it has been reduced substantially since the 1970s by successive administrative changes; and very large numbers of unemployed people have moved out of 'unemployment' into other categories, particularly sickness. (Webster, 2002)

References

Morris, J., Dangour, A., Deeming, C., Fletcher, A. and Wilkinson, P. (2005) *Minimum income for healthy living: Older people*, London: Age Concern.

Morris, J.N., Donkin, A., Wonderling, D., Wilkinson, P. and Dowler, E. (2000) 'A minimum income for healthy living', *Journal of Epidemiology and Community Health*, vol 54, pp 885-9.

Webster, D. (2002) 'Unemployment: how official statistics distort analysis and policy, and why', *Radical Statistics*, vol 79/80, Summer/Winter (www.radstats.org.uk).

Further reading

Levitas, R. and Guy, W. (eds) (1996) *Interpreting official statistics*, London: Routledge.

Weblinks

Department for Work and Pensions:
www.dwp.gov.uk

See also: 2.16 Income; 2.20 Indices of Deprivation 2004 (income domain)

2.3 Breadline Britain and the Millennium Survey of Poverty and Social Exclusion

The Breadline Britain Surveys were conducted in 1983 and 1990 by MORI for London Weekend Television and the Joseph Rowntree Foundation. These surveys were the only nationally representative surveys to use a measure of 'perceived' or 'consensual' poverty, also referred to as 'normative' poverty. This is based on the ideas of Peter Townsend (1979) regarding the definition of poverty, and means that the measure takes into account what people themselves understand and experience as the minimum acceptable standard of living in contemporary Britain. This covers not only the basic essentials for survival (food, clothing and so on) but also factors that enable people to participate in their roles in society.

In the 1990 Survey respondents were presented with a set of cards on each of which was written the name of a different item, for example, a television, a night out once a fortnight or a warm waterproof coat. Respondents were asked to place the 44 cards into one of two boxes. Box A was for items that they considered necessary – those items that all adults should be able to afford and that they should not have to do without. Box B was for items that they considered to be desirable but not necessary. They were also asked if they felt differently about any of the items in the case of families with children. An item was deemed to be a socially perceived necessity if more than 50% of respondents put it into Box A. Later in the interview the respondents were asked to assign one of the following five options to each of the 44 items, with reference to themselves:

1. Have and couldn't do without
2. Have and could do without
3. Don't have and don't want
4. Don't have and can't afford
5. Not applicable/don't know

Respondents (and their households) were assigned a Deprivation Index score each time they answered 'Don't have and can't afford' to an item that was considered to be a necessity by more than 50% of respondents (Gordon and Pantazis, 1997).

The Breadline Britain Surveys have subsequently been used in combination with census data to estimate the numbers of poor children and poor households within certain communities or areas, creating the Breadline Britain score. For the 1990 Survey, poor households were defined as those lacking ('Don't have and can't afford') at least three necessities, as described above. Data from the Survey were then related to comparable data from the 1991 Census to estimate the number of poor households in areas across Britain.

This is done by obtaining weightings for the best subset of deprivation indicator variables that were measured in both the 1991 Census and the Breadline Britain Survey, and using the multivariate statistical technique of logistic regression. This gives the best subset of (weighted) census variables that can be used as proxies of poverty. The six variables that are included are: unemployment, lack of owner-occupied accommodation and lack of car ownership, and three 'at risk' variables: limiting long-term illness, lone-parent households and low social class. The Breadline Britain score is obtained by summing the individually weighted variables and provides an estimate of the percentage of the 'poor' households in an area.

In 1999 the Millennium Survey of Poverty and Social Exclusion updated the earlier Breadline Britain Survey (Pantazis et al, 2005). Once again a representative sample of the population of Britain was asked for their views on what constitutes the necessities of life in present-day Britain. The aims of the Poverty and Social Exclusion Survey were: to update the Breadline Britain Surveys; to estimate the size of groups of households in different circumstances; to explore movement in and out of poverty; and to look at age and gender difference in experiences of and responses to poverty. The main topics covered included housing, health, time poverty, social networks and support, necessities, finance and debts, intra-household poverty, poverty over time, absolute and overall poverty, area deprivation, local services, crime, child's school, perceptions of poverty, activism as well as some demographics and information on income. The Poverty and Social Exclusion Survey additionally includes elements of social exclusion – indicating participation in social, economic, cultural and political systems and how important these are to people. It is arguably the most comprehensive survey of poverty and social exclusion ever to be undertaken in Britain.

Strengths

The main strength of the Breadline Britain measure of poverty is that it is derived not from an arbitrary cut-off point defined by government or statisticians, but by the population being studied – it thereby tells us what people themselves consider to be poverty. The ease of the interpretation of the Breadline Britain score (for example, 23% of households in a certain area live in poverty using this measure) as opposed to the use of rankings or standardised scores is also an advantage.

Limitations

A limitation of this consensual measure of poverty is that it can only truly be applied to the specific population and time period for which it was collected. Other populations will have their own understanding of what constitutes poverty, and definitions will change over time – what is a luxury for one generation may become a necessity for another. The Survey thus needs to be updated regularly in order to maintain its currency. As with some other indices (such as the English Index of Multiple Deprivation 2004), the Breadline Britain measure uses a health indicator as one of its components. It can therefore be theoretically problematic if the Breadline Britain score is used to look at associations between poverty and health, although in practice it makes little difference if the score is recalculated without the health indicator (Shaw et al, 1999).

References

Gordon, D. and Pantazis, C. (eds) (1997) *Breadline Britain in the 1990s*, Aldershot: Ashgate.

Pantazis, C., Gordon, D. and Levitas, R. (eds) (2005) *Poverty and social exclusion in Britain: The Millennium Survey*, Bristol: The Policy Press.

Shaw, M., Dorling, D., Gordon, D. and Davey Smith, G. (1999) *The widening gap: Health inequalities and policy in Britain*, Bristol: The Policy Press.

Townsend, P. (1979) *Poverty in the United Kingdom*, Harmondsworth: Penguin.

See also: 1.1 Deprivation; 2.20 Indices of Deprivation 2004; 1.10 Poverty; 2.30 Townsend Index of Deprivation

2.4 Cambridge Social Interaction and Stratification Scale (CAMSIS)

The Cambridge Social Interaction and Stratification Scale (CAMSIS) is a measure of social stratification and is usually referred to as the 'Cambridge Scale' – the original scale from which CAMSIS was developed. It uses patterns of social interaction to determine the social structure and an individual's position within it, thereby providing a hierarchical measure of social distance. The distance is defined by similarities in the lifestyles, social interactions and resources that occupational groups share. For example, people working in pairs of occupations that rarely cited each other as friends were considered to belong to groups with greater social distance, whereas those pairs of occupations that frequently cited each other were considered less distant. Thus, occupations were grouped according to friendship, which gives a numerical indication of how similar (socially close) or dissimilar (socially distant) any two occupations were. More recent versions of the scale have considered the occupations of married couples, where previous versions used friendship and marriage patterns.

The Cambridge Scale is a continuous measure, although it is often categorised into groups from the most to least advantaged. As it is based on social interactions, differences in outcomes between its groups are considered to correspond to (dis)similarities in lifestyles and health behaviours.

Example
Age-adjusted odds ratio (OR) and 95% confidence interval (CI) of coronary heart disease in men according to sextiles of Cambridge Score, Health and Lifestyles Survey, UK (Chandola, 1998)

Sixth of Cambridge Score	n	OR	95% CI
I, most advantaged	467	1.00	
II	549	1.48	0.83, 2.66
III	542	1.65	0.96, 2.86
IV	675	2.07	1.20, 3.56
V	456	2.13	1.26, 3.60
VI, least advantaged	559	2.27	1.35, 3.82
Significance of change in deviance		0.002	

In this example, the Cambridge score, a continuous measure based on similarities (or distances) in lifestyles, social interactions and resources in occupations, was divided into six groups, from those occupations that are the most to those that are the least advantaged. The table shows a strong association between this measure of SEP and coronary heart disease.

Strengths

CAMSIS gives additional insight into the social structures and resources that tend to be associated with particular occupations, and adds a further dimension to measures such as occupation-based social class.

Limitations

As with other occupational social classifications, this measure attempts to summarise a complex set of social circumstances into a single measure based simply on a person's job title and the social networks that implies. However, it does have value in helping to understand a particular aspect of the social structure and its potential impacts.

References
Chandola, T., (1998) 'Social inequality in coronary heart disease: a comparison of occupational classifications', *Social Science & Medicine*, vol 47, pp 525-33.

Further reading
Bartley, M., Sacker, A., Firth, D. and Fitzpatrick, R. (1999) 'Social position, social roles and women's health in England: changing relationships 1984-1993', *Social Science & Medicine,* vol 48, pp 99-115.
Prandy, K. (1999) 'Class, stratification and inequalities in health: a comparison of the Registrar-General's Social Classes and the Cambridge Scale', *Sociology of Health & Illness*, vol 21, pp 466-84.

Weblinks
CAMSIS bibliographic review:
www.camsis.stir.ac.uk/review.html

See also: 1.14 Social class; 1.17 Social status; 2.23 National Statistics Socioeconomic Classification (NS-SEC); 2.25 Occupation-based measures; 2.26 Occupational social class – Registrar General's Social Classes (RGSC)

2.5 Car ownership and access

Car ownership and access (whether a person has access to a car or van in their household, even if they do not own it) is a commonly used asset-based indicator of socioeconomic position (SEP). Access to a car can also be classed as a household amenity and is used to indicate – or taken as a reflection of – income and wealth: money is needed to purchase a car and also to run it.

The absence of measures of income and the inclusion of questions on car ownership and access in the census (and other surveys) has made this a key measure of SEP in the UK. It has also been used as a component of a number of deprivation indices.

Strengths

It has been argued that household asset measures such as car access are better indicators of material well-being than measures based on social class or occupation-based measures (Davey Smith and Egger, 1992), because unlike those measures they do not exclude large sections of the population, such as women, the very young or old, or unemployed people. Information about income is not often collected as it is deemed to be too sensitive a question to ask people – car access on the other hand is not seen as problematic in this way. Access to a car can also be combined with other sociodemographic variables to produce further insight; for example, the number of households without access to a car but with dependent children has been used to estimate the number of households lacking a car that might actually require one (Wheeler et al, 2005).

Limitations

The meaning of car ownership can vary by country and geographical context within countries. For instance, in the US, where car ownership is very high due to poor public transport in many areas, access to a car may have less discriminatory power to elucidate SEP than in other countries. Nevertheless, even in a country like the US, lack of access to a car may be a good indicator of very low SEP and implies reliance on a poor infrastructure of public transport to carry out day-to-day activities. It is argued that in rural areas car access is not such a good indicator of low income, as even low-income households will need to run a car. In this context, those with very low incomes may still have access to or own a car. Conversely, in city centres where public transport provision is relatively good and congestion is high, people with high incomes may choose not to have cars, even though they could afford them. Moreover, as with other measures of SEP, the meaning of the measure will change over time. While access to one car in a household would have indicated an exclusive elite in the first decades of the 20th century, by the end of the century the majority of households had access to a car, and many had access to more than one, with lack of car access indicating poverty and social exclusion (see the figure below and also Ellaway et al, 2003).

Households with access to a car or a van, Great Britain (1971-96)

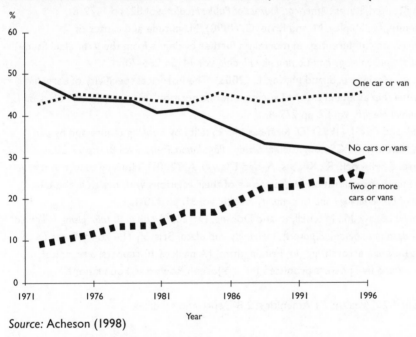

Source: Acheson (1998)

Car access and health

The relationship between car access and health is complex. Those who have access to a car have been shown to have lower mortality rates than those who do not (Filakti and Fox, 1995) even within occupational strata (Davey Smith et al, 1990). A study based on a Scottish sample looked at the relationship between access (as well as housing tenure) and various health outcomes (chronic, recent and mental health problems as well as general health), examining the effect of controlling for alternative measures of material assets – social class and income (Macintyre et al, 2001). They found that car access was still a predictor of health after controlling for social class, except for chronic illness among women. However, controlling for income considerably attenuated the association with health for most measures, indicating that car access was functioning as a measure of income. The results also suggested that car access had different implications for men and women.

References

Acheson, Sir Donald (1998) *Independent Inquiry into Inequalities in Health*, London: The Stationery Office (www.archive.official-documents.co.uk/document/doh/ih/part1b. htm).

Davey Smith, G. and Egger, M. (1992) 'Socioeconomic differences in mortality in Britain and the United States', *American Journal of Public Health*, vol 82, pp 1079-81.

Davey Smith, G., Shipley, M. and Rose, G. (1990) 'Magnitude and causes of socioeconomic differentials in mortality: further evidence from the Whitehall Study', *Journal of Epidemiology and Community Health*, vol 44, pp 265-70.

Ellaway, A., Macintyre, S. and McKay, L. (2003) 'The historical specificity of early life car ownership as an indicator of socioeconomic position', *Journal of Epidemiology and Community Health*, vol 57, pp 277-8.

Filakti, H. and Fox, J. (1995) 'Differences in mortality by housing tenure and by car access from the OPCS Longitudinal Study', *Population Trends*, vol 81, pp 27-30.

Macintyre, S., Hiscock, R., Kearns, A. and Ellaway, A. (2001) 'Housing tenure and car access: further exploration of the nature of their relations with health in the UK', *Journal of Epidemiology and Community Health*, vol 51, pp 330-1.

Wheeler, B., Shaw, M., Mitchell, R. and Dorling, D. (2005) *Life in Britain: Using millennial Census data to understand poverty, inequality and place*, Bristol: The Policy Press (www. shef.ac.uk/sasi/research/life_in_britain_.htm) [A pack of 10 reports, a technical, summary and five posters produced for the Joseph Rowntree Foundation].

See also: 1.20 Wealth; 2.1 Amenities; 2.8 Deprivation indices

2.6 Carstairs Deprivation Index

The Carstairs Deprivation Index is one of a number of indices developed to measure levels of deprivation for areas. It was developed for use in relation to health in Scotland (and has mostly been used in that context) by Vera Carstairs and Russell Morris (1991) using the 1981 Census, but has also been applied to data from the 1991 and 2001 Censuses.

As with the Townsend Index of Deprivation, this is a composite measure that combines data from a number of census variables and is designed to categorise areas on a scale of poverty to affluence. The Carstairs Deprivation Index is designed to measure material deprivation through access to material resources that provide access to "those goods and services, resources and amenities and [characteristics] of a physical environment which are customary in society" (Carstairs and Morris, 1991). The focus on material resources means that it aims to reflect income and wealth. Information on income is not readily available in the UK (it was not included in the most recent 2001 Census, despite calls from many researchers; see, for example, Dorling, 1999). Items such as car ownership are included in deprivation indices such as the Carstairs Deprivation Index as proxy measures for wealth, in the absence of better data. The census variables used in the Carstairs Index are (McLoone, 2004):

- *overcrowding:* the proportion of all people living in private households with a density of more than one person per room;
- *male unemployment:* the proportion of economically active males seeking or waiting to start work;
- *low social class:* the proportion of all people in private households with an economically active head of household in social class IV or V;
- the proportion of all people in private households that do not own a car.

These individual components are then combined, using z-scores, but no weighting or transformation, to achieve a score. These are then aggregated into seven categories of deprivation.

Strengths

The advantage of an area-based approach over an individual approach is that most events or people can be assigned to an area by means of a postcode, and linking to the socioeconomic characteristics of that area allows for the inclusion of individual records that do not contain any individual-level socioeconomic information (Carstairs, 2000). A further strength is that area measures can provide information on socioeconomic context (that is, the effect of area-level deprivation on individuals living in an area, irrespective of their individual-level socioeconomic position [SEP]; see, for example, Lawlor et al, 2005). The Carstairs Deprivation Index is very similar to the Townsend Index of Deprivation, except that Carstairs includes the proportion of all people in private households with an economically active head of household in social class IV or V (which indicates SEP) in place of the proportion of private households that are not owner-occupied (which indicates lack of wealth in particular).

Limitations

Deprivation indices such as this, which rely solely on census variables, are by definition limited to the census variables collected, and restricted by any changes in the way that census data are collected over time. Although the Carstairs Index is referred to as a measure of deprivation it is intended to classify areas on a seven-point scale from poverty to affluence, yet all the component measures relate to the poverty end of the spectrum, rather than indicating wealth. Therefore, those areas classified as 'most affluent' would perhaps be more correctly described as 'least deprived'; a subtle difference, but one that might have an impact on the interpretation and use of the index. In addition, it could be argued that the inclusion of male unemployment only is an outdated method of assessing the employment status of an area, given the current participation of women in the workforce. As with all area-based measures, the ecological fallacy is always a potential problem that is invoked.

Using the same measures over time allows for the comparison of trends, but at the same time the same measure can change its meaning over time. Car ownership, for example, once indicated affluence, whereas it has now become the norm – indeed, we might want to also consider the number of households owning two or three cars as a better indicator of affluence. By the same rationale, it is also possible that not owning a car is now a stronger indicator of material deprivation than it was in 1981. Overcrowding declined substantially between 1981 and 2001 (see the table below, which shows percentages and standard deviations for the component variables of the Carstairs Index over time), meaning that its influence on the overall index may have also changed over this period. Changes in the rate of unemployment can reflect broader economic cycles as well as the economic well-being in different areas over time, so this may also affect the nature of the index at different time periods.

Population weighted mean percentages and standard deviations for each component variable used to create the Carstairs score (1981, 1991 and 2001)

	1981		1991		2001	
	Mean	Standard deviation	Mean	Standard deviation	Mean	Standard deviation
No car ownership	41.2	18.5	33.8	17.8	25.6	14.9
Male unemploy-ment	12.5	7.3	13.0	8.4	7.9	4.6
Over-crowding	25.3	11.4	7.4	4.4	4.6	2.6
Social class IV and V	24.1	10.4	20.8	8.6	18.2	7.8

Source: Adapted from McLoone (2004)

References

Carstairs, V. (2000) 'Socio-economic factors at areal level and their relationship with health', in P. Elliott, J. Wakefield, N. Best and D. Briggs (eds) *Spatial epidemiology*, Oxford: Oxford University Press.

Carstairs, V. and Morris, R. (1991) *Deprivation and health in Scotland*, Aberdeen: Aberdeen University Press.

Dorling, D. (1999) 'Who's afraid of income inequality?', *Environment and Planning A*, Commentary, vol 31, no 4, pp 571-4.

Lawlor, D., Davey Smith, G., Patel, R. and Ebrahim, S. (2005) 'Life course socioeconomic position, area deprivation and coronary heart disease: findings from the British Women's Heart and Health Study', *American Journal of Public Health*, vol 95, pp 91-7.

McLoone, P. (2004) *Carstairs scores for Scottish postcode sectors from the 2001 Census*, Glasgow: Medical Research Council Social and Public Health Sciences Unit, University of Glasgow.

Further reading

Carstairs, V. (1995) 'Deprivation indices: their interpretation and use in relation to health', *Journal of Epidemiology and Community Health*, vol 49, supp 2, pp S3-S8.

Weblinks

Carstairs deprivation scores are available at:
  http://datalib.ed.ac.uk/EUDL/carstairs.html
  www.mimas.ac.uk/

See also: 1.1 Deprivation; 1.10 Poverty; 2.8 Deprivation indices;
  2.30 Townsend Index of Deprivation

2.7 Child poverty – the official government measure

Each country has its own definition of child poverty. International researchers often use the proportion of children below the median income (see the Innocenti Research Centre weblink below). In the UK, in 2003 the Department for Work and Pensions, after consultation with academics and other experts, set out their chosen measure of child poverty 'for the long term'. They opted for a 'tiered' approach that uses a set of interrelated indicators (or tiers) designed to capture different aspects of poverty "whilst respecting the finding of our consultation that income is at the core of people's conception of poverty. Each has significance in its own right and our objective is to make progress against all indicators" (DWP, 2003, Executive Summary). These indicators are:

- *Absolute low income:* to measure whether the poorest families are seeing their incomes rise in real terms. This will be monitored by the number of children living in families with incomes below a particular threshold that is adjusted for inflation – set for a couple with one child at £210 a week in today's terms.
- *Relative low income:* to measure whether the poorest families are keeping pace with the growth of incomes in the economy as a whole. This will be monitored by the number of children living in households below 60% of contemporary median equivalised household income.
- *Material deprivation and low income combined:* to provide a wider measure of people's living standards. This will be monitored by the number of children living in households that are both materially deprived and have an income below 70% of contemporary median equivalised income.
- Using this measure, poverty is falling when all three indicators are moving in the right direction.

Previous measures have focused on measuring the proportion of households with children that have an income 60% below the median income; this new threshold of 70% will lead to more children being defined as living in poverty, and is designed to capture more of the poverty faced by families with low disposable incomes, and the high costs (such as accommodation) that they face. In order to consider trends prior to 2003, the 60% measure may need to be used.

Discussion point

Our historic aim will be for ours to be the first generation to end child poverty, and it will take a generation. It is a 20-year mission but I believe it can be done. (Prime Minister Tony Blair in 1999)

Ten steps to a society free of child poverty

1. All political parties to commit to eradicate child poverty.
2. Poverty-proof policies – make each consistent with eradicating child poverty.
3. Uprate the combined value of Child Tax Credit and Child Benefit at least in line with the fastest growing of either prices or earnings. The element of this that is Child Benefit ought to be maximised.
4. Increase the adult payments within Income Support in line with those for children.
5. Reform the administration of tax credits and benefits – ensure they get the right amount to the right people at the right time.
6. Ensure all children have full access to the requirements – meals, uniforms and activities – of their education.
7. Provide benefit entitlements to all UK residents equally, irrespective of immigration status.
8. Work towards better jobs, not just more jobs.
9. Introduce free at the point of delivery, good quality, universal childcare.
10. Reduce the disproportionate burden of taxation on poorer families.

Source: CPAG (2005)

References

CPAG (Child Poverty Action Group) (2005) *Ten steps to a society free of child poverty: Child Poverty Action Group's manifesto to eradicate child poverty*, London: CPAG (www.cpag.org.uk).

DWP (Department for Work and Pensions) (2003) *Measuring child poverty*, London: DWP (www.dwp.gov.uk).

Further reading

Ridge, T. (2002) *Childhood poverty and social exclusion: From a child's perspective*, Bristol: The Policy Press.

Stewart, K. (2005) 'Towards an equal society? Addressing childhood poverty and deprivation', in J. Hills and K. Stewart (eds) *A more equal society? New Labour, poverty, inequality and exclusion*, Bristol: The Policy Press.

Weblinks

Innocenti Research Centre:
www.unicef-icdc.org/

See also: 1.1 Deprivation; 1.10 Poverty; 3.4 Households Below Average Income
(HBAI); 2.20 Indices of Deprivation 2004

2.8 Deprivation indices

A wide variety of deprivation indices have been produced for Britain since the 1981 Census. The general function of a deprivation index is to distil a variety of deprivation measures and proxies into a single figure, or index. This index figure may represent a 'real number', for example, the proportion of households in an area estimated to be 'deprived' or 'poor'. Alternatively, the index value may in itself be meaningless, but provides an abstract numeric measure of 'deprivation', which, for example, may be used to rank areas, or to estimate the intensity of pockets of deprivation in a wider area.

Deprivation indices have generally been calculated for small areas of the country (such as electoral wards or local authority areas) for two key purposes. First, they can produce a measure of 'area socioeconomic position (SEP)' or 'area deprivation', a summary assessment of the SEP of local populations. This can be used to investigate socioeconomic and geographical inequalities in health status and health care availability, and more general geographical variation in the SEP of populations. Second, official government deprivation indices have been constructed, largely for the purposes of prioritising resource allocation, service planning and policy development.

The key deprivation indices have detailed entries elsewhere in this book, but they are summarised below for ease of reference.

Key UK deprivation indices

Official government deprivation indices (England)[a]
1991 Index of Local Conditions (Department of the Environment)
1998 Index of Local Deprivation (Department for the Environment, Transport and the Regions)
2000 Indices of Deprivation (Department for the Environment, Transport and the Regions)
2004 Indices of Deprivation (Office of the Deputy Prime Minister)
Other deprivation indices
Carstairs Deprivation Index (first produced for Scotland using 1981 Census)
Jarman underprivileged area score (first produced for England and Wales using 1981 Census)
Townsend Index of Deprivation (first produced for England using 1981 Census)
Breadline Britain Index (this is in fact a 'relative poverty index' rather than a 'deprivation index', but it has been used in similar ways to the deprivation indices)

Note: [a] Deprivation indices for Wales, Scotland and Northern Ireland have also been produced at various times using similar methods to the English Indices of Deprivation 2000/04. The indices are not generally comparable between the four countries, since they are calculated separately using different indicators.

Discussion point

In our most deprived areas – chosen because they have the worst poverty, the highest unemployment and the lowest educational achievement – we created the New Deal and Neighbourhood Renewal Programmes – £4 billion pounds worth of investment. (John Prescott, speech to the 2003 Labour Party conference)

England's most disadvantaged towns and cities will be the first to benefit from a landmark public health strategy to encourage people to lead healthier lifestyles, the health secretary, John Reid, announced today. The minister said that 88 primary care trusts (PCTs) covering the most deprived areas of the country will pilot initiatives such as healthier school meals, more services to help people stop smoking, and personal NHS health trainers who offer advice on diet and exercise. (David Batty in *The Guardian*, 19 November 2004)

Further reading

Carstairs, V. and Morris, R. (1991) *Deprivation and health in Scotland*, Aberdeen: Aberdeen University Press.

Gordon, D. (1995) 'Census based deprivation indices: their weighting and validation', *Journal of Epidemiology and Community Health*, vol 49, pp S39-S44.

Gordon, D. and Pantazis, C. (eds) (1997) *Breadline Britain in the 1990s*, Aldershot: Ashgate.

Jarman, B. (1983) 'Identification of underprivileged areas', *BMJ*, vol 286, pp 1705-8.

Townsend, P., Phillimore, P. and Beattie, A. (1988) *Health and deprivation: Inequality and the North*, London: Croom Helm.

Weblinks

The Social Disadvantage Research Centre, University of Oxford created a number of the government deprivation indices:
www.apsoc.ox.ac.uk/sdrc

A review of methods for monitoring and measuring social inequality, deprivation and health inequality:
www.ihs.ox.ac.uk/sepho/publications/carrhill/

See also: 1.1 Deprivation; 1.10 Poverty; and entries for specific deprivation indices listed on previous page

2.9 Education

Education is frequently used as a generic indicator of socioeconomic position (SEP). Despite this generic use, education is thought to specifically capture the knowledge-related assets of an individual. These assets, formally indicated by qualifications, are central to accessing employment opportunities and determining a person's adult SEP. The knowledge and skills attained through education may also affect an individual's cognitive functioning, make them more receptive to health education messages, more able to communicate with and access appropriate health services, or provide the cognitive resources that affect 'time preferences' (living in the here and now versus investing in the future) for modifying risk behaviours.

Within the life course framework, education is increasingly seen as partly reflecting somebody's early life circumstances, because it captures the transition from parental to adulthood SEP, and also as a strong determinant of future employment and income. As an exposure, it reflects material, intellectual and other resources of the family of origin, begins at an early age, is influenced by access to and performance in primary and secondary school, and reaches final attainment in young adulthood for most people. Therefore, it captures some of the long-term influences of both early life circumstances on adult health and the influence of adult resources (for example, through employment opportunities) on health.

Education is either measured as a continuous or categorical variable. When using education as a continuous measure, with number of years of completed education, the assumption is that every year of education contributes similarly to the relationship between education and health. On the other hand, using education as a categorical variable, with pre-specified categories representing milestones in the educational process, assumes that completion of specific achievements is important in determining SEP.

Strengths

The widespread use of education as an indicator of SEP reflects the fact that it is relatively easy to measure in self-administered questionnaires and response rates to educational questions tend to be high, compared to other more difficult to assess measurements such as income. Importantly, it can be obtained independently of age or working circumstances.

Limitations

It is important to note that the meaning and attainment of educational level varies for different birth cohorts and in different countries. The proportion of people reaching higher levels of education has dramatically increased in many countries in recent years, particularly among women and minority ethnic groups. Older cohorts, in studies that combine several birth cohorts, will be over-represented among the lower educated groups. As an example of good practice, in a study of mortality from cardiovascular disease among women, participants were classified into low, medium or high levels of education, these categories being defined with specific relevance to their birth cohort (Beebe-Dimmer et al, 2004). A further limitation of the use of educational levels exists, particularly among minorities, for individuals who have obtained their education outside the country of residence, in a different educational regime in which indicators of education may have very different implications than within the host country. Moreover, such migrants may also experience a mismatch between their current employment and their educational attainment in their own country.

Example

Age-adjusted 21-year death rates according to age at leaving full-time education (per 10,000 person years)

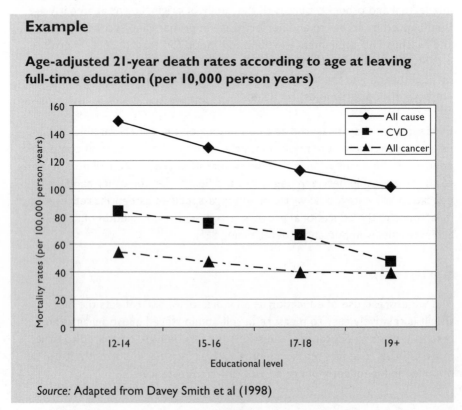

Source: Adapted from Davey Smith et al (1998)

References

Beebe-Dimmer, J., Lynch, J.W., Turrell, G., Lustgarten, S., Raghunathan, T. and Kaplan, G.A. (2004) 'Childhood and adult socioeconomic conditions and 31-year mortality risk in women', *American Journal of Epidemiology*, vol 159, pp 481-90.

Davey Smith, G., Hart, C., Hole, D., MacKinnon, P., Gillis, C., Watt, G., Blane, D. and Hawthorne, V. (1998) 'Education and occupational social class: which is the more important indicator of mortality risk?', *Journal of Epidemiology and Community Health*, vol 52, pp 153-60.

Further reading

Lynch, J. and Kaplan, G. (2000) 'Socioeconomic position', in L.F. Berkman and I. Kawachi (eds) *Social epidemiology*, Oxford: Oxford University Press, pp 13-35.

Ross, C, and Wu, C. (1995) 'The links between education and health', *American Sociological Review*, vol 60, pp 719-45.

See also: 1.7 Life course socioeconomic position

2.10 Erikson and Goldthorpe class schema

Also known as the 'Goldthorpe schema', this is an occupation-based indicator that uses employment relations to classify occupations, from jobs based on high levels of trust and independent working practices that include delegated authority, to occupations based on a labour contract with very little job control. This scheme does not have an implicit hierarchical order and therefore will not capture a gradient in health across its groups. This scheme was particularly designed to facilitate international comparisons of social stratification and mobility (Erikson and Goldthorpe, 1993).

Differences in health outcomes between groups can be attributed to differences in working relations and work autonomy, different types of contract, reward systems and terms of remuneration, and different job promotion prospects. However, the scheme also inherently reflects material resources, as decision latitude is often related to material rewards.

Strengths

This classification has a clear theoretical basis, therefore differences between groups in health outcomes can be attributed to the specific employment relations that characterise each group. In addition, construct and criterion validity of this classification have been assessed, adding to its robustness as a measure of socioeconomic position (SEP). It can be, and has been, used in international comparisons.

Limitations

Working relations and occupational circumstances are likely to change over time, and this scheme will require continuous updating. It cannot be unambiguously hierarchically ordered unless collapsed into a smaller number of categories.

Technical detail

Occupations are classified into 11 groups:

I	Service class: higher (and employers in large organisations)
IIa	Service class: lower
IIIa	Routine non-manual: higher
IIIb	Routine non-manual: lower
IVa	Small proprietors with employees
IVb	Self-employed workers in industry
IVc	Farmers/smallholders
V	Foremen and technicians
VI	Skilled manual
VIIa	Semi- and unskilled
VIIb	Agricultural workers

References

Erikson, R. and Goldthorpe, J.H. (1993) *The constant flux*, Oxford: Clarendon Press.

Further reading

Davey Smith, G. and Harding, S. (1997) 'Is control at work the key to socioeconomic gradients in mortality?', *The Lancet*, vol 350, pp 1369-70.

Kunst, A.E., Groenhof, F., Mackenbach, J.P. and Health, E.W. (1998) 'Occupational class and cause specific mortality in middle aged men in 11 European countries: comparison of population based studies', EU Working Group on Socioeconomic Inequalities in Health, *BMJ*, vol 316, pp 1636-42.

Mackenbach, J.P., Bos, V., Andersen, O. et al (2003) 'Widening socioeconomic inequalities in mortality in six Western European countries', *International Journal of Epidemiology*, vol 32, pp 830-7.

See also: 2.25 Occupation-based measures

2.11 Fuel poverty

Fuel poverty is generally defined as the inability to afford adequate home heating, or the inability to keep adequately warm at reasonable cost. The most widely accepted definition of fuel poverty is the need to spend more than 10% of household income on heating the home to an acceptable standard (Boardman, 1991). Adequate heating in the home is usually defined by World Health Organization (WHO) criteria as 21°C in the living room and 18°C in the other occupied rooms (for example, kitchen and bedrooms) (Boardman, 1991). These definitions are accepted by the UK Department of Trade and Industry (DTI) and used in current UK policy aimed at eliminating fuel poverty (DTI, 2001).

The important thing to note about the definition of fuel poverty is that it refers to how much is *needed* to heat the household adequately as opposed to how much is actually spent on heating the home. In reality many fuel-poor families are generally poor and cannot afford the amount needed to heat their homes adequately. They, thus, suffer the health and welfare effects of chronic cold exposure. Further, the amount of money needed to heat a home also takes into account the amount of time for which the home needs to be adequately heated. Thus, any households with members who do not go out to work or school (such as families with pre-school children and the retired) require more money to adequately heat their home than households where all members are out at work or school for substantial periods of time when it is considered adequate to have the house unheated or heated to a lower degree than when residents are inside. Consequently, certain groups (families with young children, the elderly, the long-term sick and disabled) are at greater risk of fuel poverty.

Causes of fuel poverty

Although fuel poverty is associated with low income it arises from the combination of low household income with inadequate and expensive forms of heating and energy inefficiency in the home. These three causes thus combine to result in fuel poverty:

- energy efficiency of the home
- fuel costs
- household income.

The solution to tackling fuel poverty therefore lies as much in capital investment, to improve the quality of housing, as it does in increasing income

(Boardman, 1991; Lawlor, 2001). This distinction from poverty in general may explain why excess winter mortality in England has not been found to be associated with standard measures of deprivation (Shah and Peacock, 1999; Lawlor et al, 2002).

Fuel poverty in the UK

It was estimated in 2000 that between four and five million households in the UK were fuel poor (Boardman, 2000). Compared to other European countries, residents from England and Ireland are more likely to report that they are unable to adequately heat their homes (Whyley and Callender, 1997). In November 2001 the government launched a policy – the UK Fuel Poverty Strategy – that has a number of targets and strategies aimed at ending the problem of fuel poverty in the UK (DTI, 2001). In particular it aims to end fuel poverty in vulnerable households (defined as any family with children, households with disabled individuals, or any household with a member who suffers a long-term illness that might be exacerbated by the cold) by 2010 and then to tackle all other households after that. The strategy focuses primarily on measures to improve energy efficiency and fuel costs for fuel-poor households, since other government initiatives are aimed at reducing income inequalities and poverty more generally.

Discussion point

Since 2003 domestic gas prices have risen by 87% and domestic electricity prices by 56%. Millions of low-income consumers and fuel poor households use prepayment meters as a way to help them budget.

But people with prepayment meters (ppms) are paying up to £173 a year more for gas and up to £113 more for electricity than quarterly billed (standard credit) consumers. (Age Concern Press Release, 4 September 2006)

Don't Pay More For The Energy You Use
Your next door neighbour could be using the same amount of gas and electricity as you, but paying a lot less because of the way he/she pays. If you pay by cash or cheque you could be paying over £100 more per year than people who pay by direct debit. Why pay more?
Change Payment Method ... be Energy Smart
(from Energywatch 'Energy Smart' leaflet)

References

Boardman, B. (1991) *Fuel poverty: From cold homes to affordable warmth*, London: Bellhaven Press.

Boardman, B. (2000) 'Resolutions for fuel poverty', *Energy Action*, February, pp 12-13.

DTI (Department of Trade and Industry) (2001) *UK Fuel Poverty Strategy* (www.dti.gov.uk)

Lawlor, D.A. (2001) 'The health consequences of fuel poverty. What should the role of primary care be?', *British Journal of General Practice*, vol 51, pp 435-6.

Lawlor, D.A., Maxwell, R. and Wheeler, B.W. (2002) 'Rurality, deprivation and excess winter mortality: an ecological study', *Journal of Epidemiology and Community Health*, vol 56, pp 373-4.

Shah, S. and Peacock, J. (1999) 'Deprivation and excess winter mortality', *Journal of Epidemiology and Community Health*, vol 53, pp 499-502.

Whyley, C. and Callender, C. (1997) *Fuel poverty in Europe – Evidence from the European Household Panel Survey, a report for NEA*, London: Policy Studies Institute.

Weblinks

Age Concern:
  www.ageconcern.org.uk
Energywatch:
  www.energywatch.org.uk

See also: 1.1 Deprivation; 1.10 Poverty

2.12 Housing conditions

Housing conditions refer to people's immediate living environment (see
2.13 Housing status and **2.14 Housing tenure**), and can be closely related
to their socioeconomic position (SEP) and also to health outcomes. These
conditions include physical features of housing, such as lighting, heating,
availability of hot water and facilities such as cooking and laundry (see
2.1 Amenities). Housing features may also extend beyond the front door,
for example for people living on the upper floors of high-rise buildings, the
presence or absence of a working lift has a major effect on living standards.
They also include consideration of the people living in the home, for example,
whether the residence is shared with other households, or if amenities such
as bathrooms or kitchens are shared. Another very important facet of housing
conditions is the degree of overcrowding (see **2.27 Overcrowding**). Lastly,
the quality of the home environment is also important, especially with regard
to problems such as ventilation, damp and infestation with insects or rodents.

Discussion point

Most people's home provides them with somewhere warm, comfortable
and safe to live. But for others it can be a nightmare from the moment
they wake up to the day's end. Damp run-down housing is causing misery
for thousands of people. (Chris Holmes, Director of Shelter, BBC Report
12/3/2002, http://news.bbc.co.uk)

Housing conditions may have a variety of impacts on the health and well-
being of householders. For example, lack of central heating has been found
to be associated with higher excess winter mortality (Aylin et al, 2001),
and cockroaches in the home have been found to produce excess asthma
symptoms in children (Rosenstreich et al, 1997).

Example

The UK census includes a variety of measures of housing condition. In
2001, residents were asked what kind of home they lived in, such as a
detached house, a flat, a bedsit, over a shop or in a caravan/mobile home.
Other questions established whether the household had sole use of,
or shared access to, a bath/shower and a toilet, whether the home had

central heating, and what the lowest floor level of the home was. In order
to ascertain whether the household shared its dwelling, the following
question was asked:

Is your household's accommodation self-contained?

This means that *all* the rooms, including the kitchen, bathroom and toilet
are behind a door that only your household can use.

- Yes, all the rooms are behind a door that only our household can use.
- No.

The exact wording of this kind of question can be important to know
when interpreting statistics from sources such as the census, especially on
indistinct concepts such as 'shared accommodation'.

The table below shows some data from the 2001 Census for England
and Wales. It demonstrates variation across some housing condition
categories in the proportion of people saying they had 'not good' general
health over the previous 12 months (as opposed to 'good' or 'fairly good'
health).

Housing conditions and general health, 2001

	Total population in household	Population with 'Not good' health	% 'not good' health
All persons	51,107,639	4,599,891	9.0
Has sole use of bath/shower and toilet	50,940,990	4,575,993	9.0
Central heating	47,289,300	4,087,508	8.6
No central heating	3,651,690	488,485	13.4
Does not have sole use of bath/shower and toilet	166,649	23,898	14.3
Central heating	119,375	15,874	13.3
No central heating	47,274	8,024	17.0

Source: Census 2001, England and Wales, Standard Table 18

References

Aylin, P., Morris, S., Wakefield, J., Grossinho, A., Jarup, L. and Elliott, P. (2001)
'Temperature, housing, deprivation and their relationship to excess winter mortality
in Great Britain, 1986-1996', *International Journal of Epidemiology*, vol 30, no 5,
pp 1100-8.

Rosenstreich, D.L., Eggleston, P., Kattan, M. et al (1997) 'The role of cockroach allergy
and exposure to cockroach allergen in causing morbidity among inner-city children
with asthma', *New England Journal of Medicine*, vol 336, pp 1356-63.

Further reading

Marsh, A., Gordon, D., Pantazis, C. and Heslop, P. (2000) *Home Sweet Home? The
impact of poor housing on health*, Bristol: The Policy Press.

Weblinks

UK census data:
  www.statistics.gov.uk
Details of the English House Conditions Survey:
  ww.communities.gov.uk/index.asp?id=1155269

See also: 2.1 Amenities; 2.13 Housing status; 2.14 Housing tenure;
  2.27 Overcrowding

2.13 Housing status (including homelessness)

The term 'housing status' can be used to refer to one of a range of aspects (or a combination of them) of housing and the area in which that housing is located. Most commonly it is used to refer to whether a person is housed, whether they are homeless, or whether they occupy some marginal status in between, such as living in temporary accommodation or staying with friends or family because they have nowhere else to go (known in the UK as 'sofa surfing') (Robinson and Coward, 2003).

Housing status can also be used to refer to the type of housing that someone occupies, common categories being whether their place of residence is a: house (detached, semi-detached, terrace); flat/apartment; rented room or bedsit; mobile home; car or van; hostel; abandoned building or squat; or they are living on the streets and sleeping rough. Another use of the term relates to whether someone lives in a private household, or in a communal establishment or institution, such as a nursing or rest home, or a university hall of residence. Housing status can also refer to how long someone has lived in their current housing, or to the amenities within that housing (such as toilets, bathrooms and cooking facilities), or the condition of the housing – whether it is in a good state of repair.

A more general use of the term relates to the area in which housing is located, for example, whether it is characterised by high-density housing, whether housing in the area is in poor condition with inadequate amenities, and at its most general, the term is used to describe the actual area lived in.

There is thus no single agreed definition of the use of this term. The measure of whether someone owns, is buying, or rents their home – their housing tenure (see **2.14**) – is far more widely (and consistently) used in the UK than housing status.

Discussion point

The Department for Communities and Local Government (DCLG) produces briefings on the English Local Authority homeless statistics four times a year.... However these releases do not reflect the true extent of homelessness in England as they only record those households that are accepted by local authorities as in priority need.

To be recorded as 'accepted' a household will have had to approach a local authority, be able to complete an application, been considered as eligible by the local authority, been recognised to be homeless and then as unintentionally homeless, and finally be accepted as in priority need.... This complex process often means that homeless people, and particularly vulnerable single homeless people, slip through the net and do not appear in official statistics on homelessness. (www.crisis.org.uk, Homelessness: information and statistics)

Homelessness

In the UK, although being homeless means not having a home, you do not have to be living on the streets to be classed as homeless. Someone may be considered legally homeless if they are:

- temporarily staying with friends or family
- staying in a hostel or bed and breakfast accommodation
- living in very overcrowded conditions
- at risk of violence or abuse in their home
- living in poor conditions that affect their health
- living somewhere that they have no legal right to stay in (for example, a squat)
- living somewhere that they cannot afford to pay for without depriving themselves of basic essentials
- forced to live apart from their family, or someone they would normally live with, because their accommodation is not suitable.

The label 'statutory homelessness' refers to those households or individuals that meet specific criteria of priority need set out in current housing legislation (such as the 2002 Homelessness Act), and to whom a homelessness duty has been accepted by a local authority. Some households/individuals will be considered to be in 'priority need', such as pregnant women or people who are vulnerable in some way. Those who are found to be 'intentionally homeless' may find that they are considered to be 'non-statutory homeless', which means their local authority has no duty to house them – this is the group most likely to be sleeping rough and whose health is most likely to suffer as a result (Shaw et al, 1999).

Homelessness is a difficult phenomenon to define and measure, and enumerations of homeless populations can be complex and controversial (Widdowfield, 1999).

References

Robinson, D. and Coward, S. (2003) *Your place, not mine: The experiences of homeless people staying with family and friends*, London: Crisis and Countryside Agency.

Shaw, M., Dorling, D. and Brimblecombe, N. (1999) 'Life chances in Britain by housing wealth and for the homeless and vulnerably housed', *Environment and Planning A*, vol 31, pp 2239-48.

Widdowfield, R. (1999) 'The limitations of official homelessness statistics', in D. Dorling and S. Simpson (eds) *Statistics in society*, London: Arnold.

Weblinks

Shelter:
www.shelter.org.uk

See also: 2.1 Amenities; 2.11 Fuel poverty; 2.14 Housing tenure; 2.27 Overcrowding

2.14 Housing tenure

Housing tenure is an asset-based measure of socioeconomic position (SEP) that refers to whether someone owns the dwelling in which they live (either outright or with a mortgage) or whether they rent it (from the public or private sector). Those who own their homes are assumed to have greater material resources and better-quality living environments than those who rent; there is evidence that they also have better health outcomes (see Example below).

Discussion point

BBC 'On this day': 20 December 1979: Council tenants will have 'right to buy'

More than five million council house tenants in Britain will be given the right to buy their home under new government proposals.

The Housing Bill published today will give tenants who have lived in their home for up to three years a 33% discount on the market value of their home, increasing in stages up to 50% for a tenancy of 20 years.

The government believes the bill will transform the social structure of Britain for good. Michael Heseltine, secretary of state for the environment, said: 'This bill lays the foundations for one of the most important social revolutions of this century'.

But Shelter, the organisation for homeless people, has said the move will increase the number of homeless people and decrease the number of homes available to accommodate them. (www.bbc.co.uk)

Strengths

Housing tenure is relatively straightforward and uncontroversial to measure. Its inclusion in the census and many other surveys means that it is widely understood and available. Apart from a small proportion of the population who may be categorised as homeless, most people can be assigned to a housing tenure category.

Limitations

Housing tenure tells us nothing of the value, size or condition of a dwelling and is therefore a very crude measure. In some rural populations, ownership of a farm, and farm size, might be more accurate measures.

The categorisation of housing tenure has changed in successive censuses, which can make comparisons over time difficult. However, careful aggregation of categories can make comparisons possible. The proportion of the population in the UK who are owner-occupiers has increased in recent years, particularly since the 'right to buy' policies of the 1980s, and 7 out of 10 households are now owner-occupied. Whereas owner-occupation used to be an indicator of high SEP, it is now more the case that renting is an indicator of low SEP.

Housing tenure in England (1918-2001)

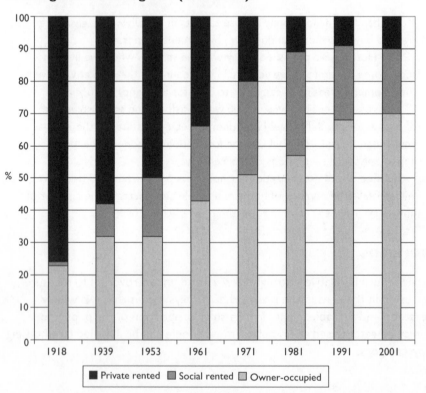

Source: Trends in tenure and cross tenure topics (general), Table S101 (www.communities.gov.uk)

Technical detail

Housing tenure classifications in the UK census
Owned outright
Owns with a mortgage or loan
Shared ownership
Rented from council
Other social rented
Private landlord or letting agency
Employer of a household member
Relative or friend of household member
Lives rent free
Not applicable (communal establishment)

Example

Housing tenure and health
Prevalence of disability in 1988, incidence and remission of disability and mortality over 15 years of follow up by gender and housing tenure

	Prevalence		Incidence		Remission		Mortality	
	Women	Men	Women	Men	Women	Men	Women	Men
Tenure	% (n)	% (n)	% (n)	% (n)	% (n)	% (n)	% (n)	% (n)
Owns/ mortgaged	24.7 (107)	19.1 (57)	4.5 (108)	3.6 (55)	6.1 (26)	5.1 (10)	10.6 (354)	13.6 (261)
Private/ council rented	31.3 (95)	24.7 (36)	5.7 (76)	4.4 (26)	3.4 (16)	4.4 (5)	12.2 (263)	17.3 (139)
Living with others/ warden assisted	40.2 (90)	36.1 (26)	5.9 (46)	5.9 (14)	3.0 (10)	6.3 (5)	15.9 (211)	17.9 (70)

Source: Adapted from Matthews et al (2006)

References

Matthews, R.J., Jagger, C. and Hancock, R.M. (2006) 'Does socio-economic advantage lead to a longer, healthier old age?', *Social Science & Medicine*, vol 62, pp 2489-99.

See also: 2.13 Housing status; 2.15 Housing wealth

2.15 Housing wealth

Housing wealth is the single most important source of personal wealth for people in the UK (Thomas and Dorling, 2004). Housing wealth refers to the amount of equity people own in their property. For those people who live in rented property and own no other property, their housing wealth is by definition zero. In the absence of other measures of wealth, and because of its importance in determining overall wealth, housing wealth is often used as a proxy for wealth more generally.

Discussion point

Wealth tied up in housing is driving a wedge between rich and poor. Those at the top of the housing ladder have seen their housing wealth increase by over 300 per cent in the last ten years alone, while those at the bottom of the ladder accumulate no housing wealth at all. (Thomas and Dorling, 2004)

Council Tax bands

One way of approximating housing wealth is to use the Council Tax bands, which came into effect in April 1993. This measure includes people living in rented accommodation and is thus not a measure of housing equity per se, but an indication of the value of the home in which a person lives, regardless of who owns that home. It can thus be considered an indicator of socioeconomic position (SEP) directly based on the housing in which a person lives.

For the purposes of Council Tax each dwelling was assigned a Council Tax band corresponding to a letter code in the range A–H (I in Wales), each representing a specific range of property market values. The basis of the valuation for a dwelling that is not used for any business purpose is the amount that, subject to certain assumptions, it would have sold for on the 'open market' by a 'willing vendor' on 1 April 1991 (1 April 2003 in Wales). All domestic property was assigned to one of these bands for the administration of Council Tax bills. There are different valuation bands in England and in Wales. More specific details of the housing characteristics that are taken into account, and the necessary assumptions to place each property into these bands, can be found on the website of the Valuation Office Agency (see Weblinks).

Technical detail – Council Tax valuation bands in England and Wales

England

Valuation band	Property market value at 1 April 1991
Band A	up to £40,000
Band B	£40,001-£52,000
Band C	£52,001-£68,000
Band D	£68,001-£88,000
Band E	£88,001-£120,000
Band F	£120,001-£160,000
Band G	£160,001-£320,000
Band H	£320,001 and above

Wales

Old bands pre 1 April 2005	Current bands with effect from 1 April 2005
Band A ... up to £30,000	Band A... up to £44,000
Band B ... £30,001-£39,000	Band B... £44,001-£65,000
Band C ... £39,001-£51,000	Band C... £65,001-£91,000
Band D ... £51,001-£66,000	Band D... £91,001-£123,000
Band E ... £66,001-£90,000	Band E... £123,001-£162,000
Band F ... £90,001-£120,000	Band F... £162,001-£223,000
Band G ... £120,001-£240,000	Band G... £223,001-£324,000
Band H ... £240,001 and above	Band H... £324,001-£424,000
	Band I... £424,001 and above

Strengths

The advantage of using a measure of housing equity is that it is a truer gauge of a person's wealth than the Council Tax bands. However, this information is much more difficult to collect and access than information on Council Tax bands. These bands are readily available from public databases, and can be assigned to each individual, contrary to other geographical indices of deprivation, which may give rise to the ecological fallacy when used to study individual SEP. Council Tax bands have been used in health research showing that this measure correlates well with individual SEP (Fone et al, 2006). In addition, higher Council Tax bands, reflecting higher housing value, have been found to be associated with lower mortality rates (Beale et al, 2002).

Limitations

Housing wealth may not always reflect income and living standards. A person can be housing-rich and income-poor. This is especially likely for older people who own their own homes, which may have increased markedly in value since they originally purchased them, but have relatively low incomes based on pensions and/or benefits. For those who own more than one property, using Council Tax bands as an indicator of housing equity will underestimate total wealth as it is based on first/main residence. Also, using Council Tax bands for England based on values in 1991 ignores subsequent uneven changes in the housing market. Fluctuations in the housing market also add difficulty here, particularly in comparisons over time.

Example

Mortality rates and 95% confidence intervals in a UK general practice in 1999

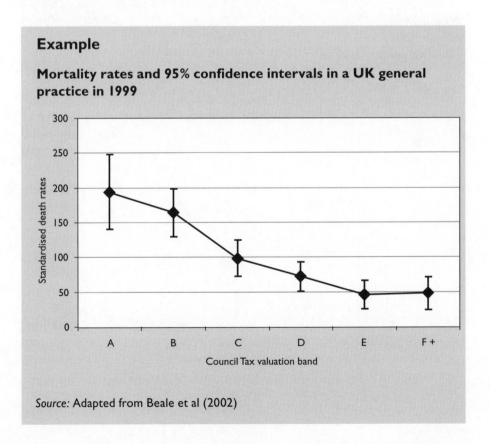

Source: Adapted from Beale et al (2002)

References

Beale, N., Taylor, G. and Straker-Cook, D. (2002) 'Is council tax valuation band a predictor of mortality?', *BMC Public Health*, vol 2, article 17 (www.biomedcentral.com/1471-2458/2/17).

Fone, D., Dunstan, F., Christie, S., Jones, A., West, J., Webber, M., Lester, N. and Watkins, J. (2006) 'Council tax valuation bands, socio-economic status and health outcome: a cross-sectional analysis from the Caerphilly Health and Social Needs Study', *BMC Public Health*, vol 6, article 115 (www.biomedcentral.com/1471-2458/6/115).

Thomas, B. and Dorling, D. (2004) *Know your place: Housing wealth and inequality in Great Britain 1980-2003 and beyond*, London: Shelter.

Further reading

Shaw, M., Dorling, D. and Brimblecombe, N. (1999) 'Life chances in Britain by housing wealth and for the homeless and vulnerably housed', *Environment and Planning A*, vol 31, pp 2239-48.

Weblinks

Valuation Office Agency:
www.voa.gov.uk/index.htm

See also: 1.20 Wealth; 2.14 Housing tenure; 4.8 Ecological fallacy

2.16 Income

Income is the indicator of socioeconomic position (SEP) that most directly measures material resources. As with other indicators such as education, income has a 'dose-response' association with health. Income also has a cumulative effect over the life course and is the SEP indicator that can change most on a short-term basis, although this dynamic aspect is rarely taken into account in epidemiological studies.

Individuals can either be asked to report their absolute income or asked to place themselves within predefined categories. Individual income will capture individual material characteristics, whereas household income may be a more useful indicator, particularly for women, who have not traditionally been the main earners in the household. Using household income information to apply to all the individuals in the household assumes an even distribution of income according to needs within the household, which may or may not be true. For income to be comparable across households, additional information on family size or the number of people dependent on the reported income should be elicited. This can be then transformed into 'equivalised income', which adjusts for family size and its associated costs of living.

Income can influence a wide range of material circumstances with direct implications for health, although it is implausible that money per se directly affects health. Thus it is the conversion of money and assets into health-enhancing commodities and services via expenditure that might be the more relevant concept for understanding how income affects health. Consumption measures are, however, rarely used in epidemiological studies.

Income primarily influences health through a direct effect on material resources that are in turn mediated by more proximal factors in the causal chain. For example, buying access to better-quality material resources such as food and shelter; allowing access to services that may enhance health directly (such as health services, leisure activities) or indirectly (such as education); fostering self-esteem and social standing by providing the outward material characteristics relevant to participation in society. Income may also affect health-related behaviours (smoking, compliance with treatment for chronic disease and so on). Reverse causality (that is, health status affecting income) should also be considered, as income level changes throughout the life course and can be affected by health status.

Discussion point

If we made an income pyramid out of a child's blocks, with each layer portraying $1,000 of income, the peak would be far higher than the Eiffel Tower, but almost all of us would be within a yard of the ground. (Paul Samuelson, winner of the Nobel Prize in Economics, 1948)

By the end of the century, Samuelson found that although there would be some modest alterations at the bottom, the world had changed so much the peak would be as high as Mount Everest. (Alperovitz, 2005)

Strengths

Income is arguably the most direct single indicator of material living standards.

Limitations

There is evidence that personal income is a sensitive issue and people may be reluctant to provide such information. Ideally we want to collect data on disposable income as this reflects what individuals/households can actually spend, but often we measure gross incomes or incomes that do not take account of in-kind transfers that function as hypothecated income (such as Food Stamps in the US). The meaning of current income for different age groups may vary and be most sensitive during the prime earning years. Income for young and older adults may be a less reliable indicator of their true SEP because income typically follows a curvilinear trajectory with age. Income can often be confused with wealth; they are usually related, but not always. Someone may be very wealthy with a low income, or conversely may have a high income but little accumulated wealth.

Example

Age-adjusted prevalence (%) of poor self-rated health in the Whitehall II Study

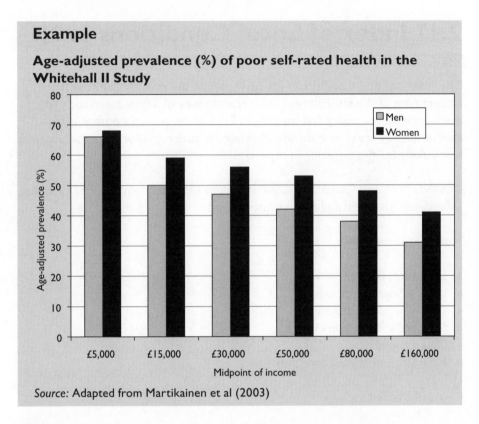

Source: Adapted from Martikainen et al (2003)

References

Alperovitz, G. (2005) 'Taking the offensive on wealth', *The Nation*, 21 February.

Martikainen, P., Adda, J., Ferrie, J.E., Davey Smith, G. and Marmot, M. (2003) 'Effects of income and wealth on GHQ depression and poor self rated health in white collar women and men in the Whitehall II study', *Journal of Epidemiology and Community Health*, vol 57, pp 718-23.

Further reading

Ecob, R. and Davey Smith, G. (1999) 'Income and health: what is the nature of the relationship?', *Social Science & Medicine*, vol 48, no 5, pp 693-705.

Krieger, N., Williams, D.R. and Moss, N.E. (1997) 'Measuring social class in US public health research: concepts, methodologies, and guidelines', *Annual Review of Public Health*, vol 18, pp 341-78.

Weblink

The Whitehall II Study:
www.ucl.ac.uk/whitehallII

See also: 1.10 Poverty; 1.20 Wealth; 2.15 Housing wealth

2.17 Index of Local Conditions 1991

The Index of Local Conditions was developed in the mid-1990s by the then Department of the Environment as a general index of urban deprivation to assist government policy and planning in England. Its main purpose was to be able to identify areas with the greatest need in order to allocate resources, and particularly for the targeting of regeneration.

The Index of Local Conditions used data from 1991 and comprised 13 variables, six non-census-based and seven census-based.

Non-census variables:

- Long-term unemployment
- Income Support recipients
- Low educational attainment
- Standardised mortality ratios
- Derelict land
- House contents insurance premiums

Census variables:

- Unemployment
- Children in low-earning households
- Overcrowding
- Housing lacking basic amenities
- Lack of car ownership
- Children in 'unsuitable' accommodation
- Educational participation at age 17

The Index is calculated as an unweighted summation of the selected indicators using their log-transformed signed chi-square values. All indicators hold equal weight in the index. Scores greater then 0 indicate greater levels of material deprivation. At the electoral ward level, only the census-based variables are used in the calculation of the index.

Because the Index of Local Conditions can be expressed as a ranked score it has been particularly useful for comparisons between small areas and between local authorities. The indicators that comprise the Index were chosen as they derive from robust data sets and span a range of aspects of deprivation. It was criticised by some for not including ethnicity but others argue that ethnicity should not have been included as it is not a direct measure of deprivation per se. As one of the component indicators is a health measure (standardised mortality ratios [SMRs]), again not a direct indicator of deprivation, it can be argued that analyses of the association between the Index and measures of mortality should not be performed as they will necessarily be correlated to some degree.

Example

Deprivation and health
A study of 107 local education authority areas in 1991 looked at the relationship between educational attainment at age 15/16, the Index of Local Conditions and mortality. Educational attainment was found to be closely associated with all cause, coronary, and infant mortality and strongly associated with the Index of Local Conditions. This social index was also closely associated with all the measures of mortality. In multiple regression analyses, the local conditions index was the stronger correlate of all cause mortality but for coronary and infant mortality, educational attainment remained highly statistically significant. The authors concluded that area levels of both educational attainment and deprivation-affluence are strong correlates of local mortality rates in England. (Morris et al, 1996)

The Index of Local Conditions was superseded by the Department for the Environment, Transport and the Regions' deprivation indices.

References
Morris, J., Blane, D. and White, I. (1996) 'Levels of mortality, education, and social conditions in the 107 local education authority areas of England', *Journal of Epidemiology and Community Health*, vol 50, pp 15-17.

See also: 1.1 Deprivation; 2.8 Deprivation indices; 2.18 Index of Local Deprivation 1998; 2.19 and 2.20 Indices of Deprivation 2000 and 2004

2.18 Index of Local Deprivation 1998

This is an area-level deprivation measure (see **2.8 Deprivation indices**). The Department for the Environment, Transport and the Regions' Index of Local Deprivation (1998) superseded the Department of the Environment's Index of Local Conditions (1991). This new indicator was an update of the previous index and based mainly on data from 1996. It was calculated for the 354 English local authorities as they existed in April 1998 and contains 12 component indicators (with year of data used shown in brackets):

- Unemployment (1997)
- Dependent children of Income Support recipients (1996)
- Overcrowding (1991 Census)
- Housing lacking basic amenities (1991 Census)
- Non-Income Support recipients in receipt of Council Tax benefit (1996)
- Educational participation (1991 Census)
- Long-term unemployment (1997)
- Income Support (1996)
- Low educational attainment (1996)
- Standardised mortality ratios (1996)
- Derelict land (1993)
- Home insurance weightings (1996)

In this 1998 Index only the positive values (those where the actual count exceeds that expected) are summed whereas for the 1991 Index of Local Conditions the values for the indicators are added together to produce the overall index score. Also, the 1991 Index did not include any weightings, while for the 1998 Index the values for the standardised mortality ratio (SMR) and home insurance premium indicators are multiplied by two, increasing the influence of these indicators on the final index.

This Index of Local Deprivation was superseded by the Department for the Environment, Transport and the Regions' Indices of Local Deprivation (2000).

Weblinks
Department of Communities and Local Government:
  www.communities.gov.uk/index.asp?id=1128648

See also: 1.1 Deprivation; 2.8 Deprivation indices; 2,17 Index of Local Conditions 1991; 2.19 and 2.20 Indices of Deprivation 2000 and 2004

2.19 Indices of Deprivation 2000

The Indices of Deprivation 2000 are area-level measures of deprivation consisting of:

- Separate indices at ward level on each of *six domains*:
  1. Income (25%)
  2. Employment (25%)
  3. Health deprivation and disability (15%)
  4. Education skills and training (15%)
  5. Housing (10%)
  6. Geographical access to services (10%)

  This allows all 8,414 wards in England to be ranked according to how deprived they are relative to other wards, for each domain. The percentages in parentheses show weights for the Index of Multiple Deprivation (IMD), with the most robust domains having the most weight. Several measures were produced using these domains:

- A ward-level index that brings together the six domains of deprivation into one overall *Index of Multiple Deprivation*, known as the IMD 2000.
- A supplementary *Child Poverty Index* at ward level that gives the percentage of children living in households that claim means-tested benefits.
- Six *district level summaries* of the IMD 2000 that allow all 354 local authority districts to be ranked according to each measure. These summaries take account of the different patterns of deprivation found in different areas. These six summary measures are: local concentration, extent, income scale, employment scale, average score and average rank.

'Average score' is the population-weighted average of the combined scores for the wards in a local authority whereas 'average rank' is the population-weighted average of the combined ranks for the wards in a local authority.

These indices were produced after a review by the University of Oxford, commissioned by the Department for the Environment, Transport and the Regions, of the 1998 Index of Local Deprivation. This review took into account previous criticisms and newly available and more up-to-date data. Indicators were selected for which there were statistically robust data available at small area level for the whole of England. They were also selected as direct indicators of deprivation.

'Hot spots' of deprivation can be identified by 'local concentration', which is the population-weighted average of the ranks of a district's most deprived wards that contain exactly 10% of the district's population. How widespread high levels of deprivation are in a district can be measured by 'extent', which is the proportion of a district's population living in the wards that rank within the most deprived 10% of wards in the country. Two measures of 'scale' are designed to give an indication of the sheer numbers of people experiencing income deprivation and employment deprivation. 'Income scale' is the number of people who are income deprived; 'employment scale' is the number of people who are employment deprived. These are absolute measures and therefore cannot be used to compare areas without considering additional factors.

Strengths

The 2000 Indices are based on a much broader range of indicators than their predecessors (see box below). The advantage of having the six separate domains means that each type of deprivation in an area can be described. Also, analyses can be conducted with components of the IMD as well as with the composite index. For example, if the research question involves looking at patterns of health, then because the IMD contains a measure of this it is not ideal to use it in this form but better to use the other individual domains.

Limitations

One issue with the combined IMD 2000 score that uses all six domains is that the 'geographical access to services' domain behaves quite differently to the others. In general, the other five domains are positively associated with each other – for example, areas that are income deprived tend also to be employment deprived. However, the access domain is negatively associated with the other five indicators, and also with the IMD itself. This means that areas that are more 'access deprived' tend to be less deprived on all the other domains. This can be explained by the fact that deprivation (in terms of income, education and so on) is largely concentrated in central urban areas, which actually have very good geographical access to services, since GP surgeries, post offices and so on are likely to be a relatively small distance away. This is contrasted with rural and suburban areas that in general tend to be less deprived, but are at a greater distance from these kinds of services. While the IMD and the access domain are still useful, this anomaly may be of some importance in certain circumstances.

Domains and indicators of the Indices of Deprivation 2000

Income deprivation

This domain measures people on a low income; these are non-overlapping counts of people in families in receipt of means-tested benefits.

Adults in Income Support households (DSS) 1998
Children in Income Support households (DSS) 1998
Adults in Income-based Jobseeker's Allowance households (DSS) 1998
Children in Income-based Jobseeker's Allowance households (DSS) 1998
Adults in Family Credit households (DSS) 1999
Children in Family Credit households (DSS) 1999
Adults in Disability Working Allowance households (DSS) 1999
Children in Disability Working Allowance households (DSS) 1999
Non-earning, non-Income Support pensioner and disabled Council Tax
    Benefit recipients (DSS) 1998, apportioned to wards

Employment deprivation

This domain measures forced exclusion from the world of work – people who want to work but are unable to do so because of unemployment, sickness or disability.

Unemployment claimant counts (JUVOS, ONS) average of May 1998,
    August 1998, November 1998 and February 1999
People out of work but in Training and Enterprise Council (TEC) delivered
    government-supported training (DfEE)
People aged 18-24 on New Deal options (ES)
Incapacity Benefit recipients aged 16-59 (DSS) 1998
Severe Disablement Allowance claimants aged 16-59 (DSS) 1999

Health deprivation and disability

This domain identifies people whose quality of life is impaired by either poor health or disability.

Comparative mortality ratios for men and women at ages under 65. District
    level figures for 1997 and 1998 applied to constituent wards (ONS)
People receiving Attendance Allowance or Disability Living Allowance (DSS)
    1998, as a proportion of all people
Proportion of people of working age (16-59) receiving Incapacity Benefit or
    Severe Disablement Allowance (DSS) 1998 and 1999 respectively

Age and sex-standardised ratios of limiting long-term illness (1991 Census)
Proportion of births of low birth weight (<2,500g) (ONS) 1993-97

Education, skills and training deprivation
This domain measures education deprivation in as direct a way as
possible, predominantly through lack of qualifications.

Working-age adults with no qualifications (three years aggregated LFS data
   at district level, modelled to ward level) 1995-98
Children aged 16 and over who are not in full-time education (Child Benefit
   data – DSS) 1999
Proportions of population aged 17-19 who have not successfully applied for
   Higher Education (UCAS data) 1997 and 1998
Key Stage 2 primary school performance data (DfEE, converted to ward
   level estimates) 1998
Primary school children with English as an additional language (DfEE) 1998
Absenteeism at primary level (all absence, not just unauthorised) (DfEE)
   1998

Housing deprivation
This domain identifies people living in unsatisfactory housing, and in the
extreme case, homelessness.

Homeless households in temporary accommodation (local authority
   Housing Improvement Programme [HIP] returns) 1997-98
Household overcrowding (1991 Census)
Poor private sector housing (modelled from 1996 English House Condition
   Survey and RESIDATA)

Geographical access to services
This domain focuses on access to essential services for people on
benefits.

Access to a post office (General Post Office Counters) April 1998
Access to food shops (Data Consultancy) 1998
Access to a GP (NHS, BMA, Scottish Health Service) October 1997
Access to a primary school for all 5- to 8-year-olds (DfEE) 1999

Child Poverty Index
This is a subset of the Income Domain Index; it is not combined with the other domains in the overall IMD as child poverty is already captured in the income domain.

Percentage of children in each ward who live in families that claim means-tested benefits (Income Support, Jobseeker's Allowance [income-based], Family Credit and Disability Working Allowance)

Source: DETR (Department of the Environment, Transport and the Regions) (2000) *Indices of Deprivation 2000*, Regeneration Research Summary Number 31, London: DETR (www.communities.gov.uk/pub/632/IndicesofDeprivation2000summaryPDF158Kb_id1128632.pdf).

The Indices of Deprivation 2000 were superseded by the Indices of Deprivation 2004.

Weblinks
Information on these indices at the Communities and Local Government website:
www.communities.gov.uk/index.asp?id=1128626
Ward level data:
www.neighbourhood.statistics.gov.uk

See also: 1.1 Deprivation; 2.8 Deprivation indices; 2.18 Index of Local Deprivation 1998; 2.20 Indices of Deprivation 2004

2.20 Indices of Deprivation 2004

The English Indices of Deprivation 2004 are area-level measures of deprivation that superseded the Indices of Deprivation 2000. They are based on the same approach and methodology but have been revised using some updated data sources and some new and improved data sources. The Indices of Deprivation 2004 contain a total of 37 indicators, compared to 33 in the Indices of Deprivation 2000, and seven rather than six domains. The indicators were chosen on the following criteria: they should measure deprivation as directly as possible and be domain-specific; they should measure major features of deprivation not just conditions experienced by a small minority; they should be up-to-date and capable of being updated on a regular basis; they should be statistically robust and available for the whole of England at a small area level on a consistent basis.

- The *seven domains* of the Indices of Deprivation 2004 are:
  1. Income (22.5%)
  2. Employment (22.5%)
  3. Health and disability (13.5%)
  4. Education, skills and training (13.5%)
  5. Barriers to housing and services (9.3%)
  6. Living environment (9.3%)
  7. Crime (9.3%).

Rather than for wards the Indices of Deprivation 2004 are calculated for 32,482 super output areas (SOAs) in England. The percentages show weights for the Index of Multiple Deprivation (IMD), with the most robust domains having the most weight.

- The seven domains are brought together into one overall *Index of Multiple Deprivation* known as the IMD 2004. The overall IMD is conceptualised as a weighted area level aggregation of the specific dimensions of deprivation. Each SOA is assigned a *score* and a *rank* for the IMD 2004.
- Six summary measures are used to reflect different patterns of deprivation. These are the same as for the Indices of Deprivation 2000 (average of SOA ranks; average of SOA scores; local concentration; extent; income scale; employment scale).

The indices use the same methodology, and similar data to those for 2000 are subject to the same strengths and limitations.

Domains and indicators of the Indices of Deprivation 2004

Income deprivation

The purpose of this domain is to capture the proportion of the population experiencing income deprivation in an area.

Adults and children in Income Support households 2001 (DWP)

Adults and children in Income-based Jobseeker's Allowance households 2001 (DWP)

Adults and children in Working Families Tax Credit households whose equivalised income (excluding Housing Benefit) is below 60% of median before housing costs 2001 (Inland Revenue)

Adults and children in Disabled Person's Tax Credit households whose equivalised income (excluding Housing Benefit) is below 60% of median before housing costs 2001 (Inland Revenue)

National Asylum Support Service supported asylum seekers in England in receipt of subsistence only and accommodation support 2002 (Home Office and National Asylum Support Service)

In addition, an Income Deprivation Affecting Children Index and an Income Deprivation Affecting Older People Index were created.

Employment deprivation

This domain measures employment deprivation conceptualised as involuntary exclusion of the working-age population from the world of work.

Unemployment claimant count (JUVOS) of women aged 18-59 and men aged 18-64 averaged over four quarters 2001 (ONS)

Incapacity Benefit claimants women aged 18-59 and men aged 18-64, 2001

Severe Disablement Allowance claimants women aged 18-59 and men aged 18-64, 2001 (DWP)

Participants in New Deal for the 18-24s who are not included in the claimant count 2001 (DWP)

Participants in New Deal for 25+ who are not included in the claimant count 2001 (DWP)

Participants in New Deal for Lone Parents aged 18 and over 2001 (DWP)

Health deprivation and disability

This domain identifies areas with relatively high rates of people who die prematurely or whose quality of life is impaired by poor health or who are disabled, across the whole population.

Years of potential life lost 1997-2001 (ONS)
Comparative illness and disability ratio 2001 (DWP, ONS)
Measures of emergency admissions to hospital 1999-2002 (DH)
Adults under 60 suffering from mood or anxiety disorders 1997-2002 (DH)

Education, skills and training deprivation
This domain captures the extent of deprivation in terms of education,
skills and training in a local area. The indicators fall into two subdomains:
one relating to education deprivation for children/young people in
the area and one relating to lack of skills and qualifications among the
working-age adult population.

Subdomain: Children/young people
Average points score of children at Key Stage 2, 2002 (DfES)
Average points score of children at Key Stage 3, 2002 (DfES)
Average points score of children at Key Stage 4, 2002 (DfES)
Proportion of young people *not* staying on in school or school-level
education above 16, 2001 (DfES)
Proportion of those aged under 21 not entering higher education
1999-2002 (UCAS)
Secondary school absence rate 2001-02 (DfES)

Subdomain: Skills
Proportions of working-age adults (aged 25-54) in the area with no or
low qualifications 2001 (ONS)

Barriers to housing and services
The purpose of this domain is to measure barriers to housing and key
local services. The indicators fall into two subdomains: 'geographical
barriers' and 'wider barriers', which also includes issues relating to access
to housing, such as affordability.

Subdomain: Wider barriers
Household overcrowding 2001 (ONS)
Local authority level percentage of households for whom a decision on
their application for assistance under the homeless provisions of housing
legislation has been made, assigned to SOAs, 2002 (ODPM)
Difficulty of access to owner-occupation 2002 (Heriot-Watt University)

Subdomain: Geographical barriers
Road distance to GP premises 2003 (NHSIA)

Road distance to a supermarket or convenience store 2002 (MapInfo Ltd)
Road distance to a primary school 2001-02 (DfES)
Road distance to a post office 2003 (Post Office Ltd)

Crime

This domain measures the incidence of recorded crime for four major
crime themes, representing the occurrence of personal and material
victimisation at a small area level.

Burglary (four recorded crime offence types) April 2002-March 2003
 (Home Office)
Theft (five recorded crime offence types) April 2002-March 2003,
 constrained to CDRP level (Home Office)
Criminal damage (10 recorded crime offence types) April 2002-March 2003
 (Home Office)
Violence (14 recorded crime offence types) April 2002-March 2003
 (Home Office)

Living environment deprivation

This domain focuses on deprivation with respect to the characteristics of
the living environment. It comprises two subdomains: the 'indoors' living
environment that measures the quality of housing, and the 'outdoors'
living environment that contains two measures about air quality and road
traffic accidents.

Subdomain: 'Indoors' living environment
Social and private housing in poor condition 2001 (ODPM)
Houses without central heating 2001 (ONS)

Subdomain: 'Outdoors' living environment
Air quality 2001 (Staffordshire University)
Road traffic accidents involving injury to pedestrians and cyclists 2000-02

Source: Indices of Deprivation 2004: summary (revised)
(www.communities.gov.uk/index.asp?id=1128444)

See also: 1.1 Deprivation; 2.8 Deprivation indices; 2.19 Indices of Deprivation 2000;
 2.24 Northern Ireland Multiple Deprivation Measure (NIMDM) 2005;
 2.29 Scottish Index of Multiple Deprivation (SIMD) 2004;
 2.32 Welsh Index of Multiple Deprivation (WIMD) 2005

2.21 Jarman underprivileged area (UPA) score

The Jarman, or underprivileged area (UPA), score was originally designed to measure the demand for primary healthcare in terms of general practitioner (GP) workloads (and was used to calculate GP payments). However, it is often taken to be a reflection of 'social deprivation'. It is a composite score (sometimes referred to as UPA8) that can be calculated for areas and is based on census data; it includes the following census variables:

1. *Unemployment:* unemployed residents aged 16+ as a proportion of all economically active residents aged 16+. (3.34)
2. *Overcrowding:* people in households with one or more people per room as a proportion of all residents in households. (2.88)
3. *Lone pensioners:* lone-pensioner households as a proportion of all residents in households. (6.62)
4. *Single parents:* lone parents as a proportion of all residents in households. (3.01)
5. *Born in New Commonwealth:* residents born in the New Commonwealth or Pakistan as a proportion of all residents. (2.5)
6. *Children aged under five:* children aged 0-4 years of age as a proportion of all residents. (4.64)
7. *Low social class:* people in households with economically active head of household in socioeconomic group 11 (unskilled manual workers) as a proportion of all people in households. (3.74)
8. *One-year migrants:* residents with a different address one year before the census as a proportion of all residents. (2.68)

These eight factors and weights (shown in brackets above) were originally derived from a survey of GPs of what population characteristics contributed most to their workload. In order to derive a single figure index using these eight factors, the arcsine of the square root of each variable is calculated, and Z scores are summed according to these weights. The average score for the nation is set at 0, with a score above 0 reflecting relatively high needs, and a score below 0 indicating relatively low needs. A score of over 30 is considered to have the highest health needs, and GP practices with scores higher than 30 receive an additional 'deprivation payment' for the workload they will incur.

Strengths

The Jarman UPA score is multidimensional and widely used in the NHS. As it is based on census data, the score can be calculated for all electoral wards (as the score was originally calculated) or enumeration districts (as it has been calculated since April 1999).

Limitations

Although there is a strong link between deprivation and the need for healthcare, the Jarman UPA score should be used with caution as an 'all-purpose' indicator of deprivation. It is designed specifically to reflect the influence of population characteristics on GP workload, rather than as a general index of material deprivation. Some of the composite variables are purely demographic (such as children aged under five) and do not necessarily indicate deprivation per se. Also, census data are collected only every 10 years, and there may be under-enumeration in the census of some groups with high levels of healthcare need (and deprivation) such as homeless people or asylum seekers. Changing patterns of migration may also have an impact on GP workloads that the New Commonwealth category does not adequately reflect.

A study comparing the Townsend, Carstairs and Jarman Indices as predictors of GP workload found that the Townsend Index was the best predictor (Ben-Shlomo et al, 1992). The overcrowding and geographical mobility variables used in the Jarman Index did not predict increased workload and the weighting assigned to children under five under-estimated the additional workload this group generated. The study concluded that other indices that include car ownership and housing tenure are better predictors of GP workload. The Jarman UPA score has also been criticised for being a better reflection of inner-city than of rural deprivation (Davies, 1998) because of the inclusion of overcrowding and ethnicity.

References
Ben-Shlomo, Y., White, I. and McKeigue, P. (1992) 'Prediction of general practice workload from census based social deprivation scores', *Journal of Epidemiology and Community Health*, vol 46, pp 532-6.
Davies, J. (1998) 'Healthy Living Centres', *Health Services Journal*, November, pp 1-5.

Further reading
Davey Smith, G. (1991) 'Second thoughts on the Jarman index', *BMJ*, vol 302, pp 359-60.

Jarman, B. (1983) 'Identification of underprivileged areas', *BMJ*, vol 286, pp 1705-8.
Jarman, B. (1984) 'Underprivileged areas: validation and distribution of scores', *BMJ*, vol 289, pp 1587-92.

See also: 1.1 Deprivation; 2.6 Carstairs Deprivation Index; 2.8 Deprivation indices; 2.30 Townsend Index of Deprivation

2.22 Job insecurity

In addition to the type of work undertaken, and whether and for how long an individual is unemployed, attention has also recently focused on the issue of job (in)security, reflecting changes in working conditions.

'Job insecurity' refers to whether a person feels that their job, or a certain valued condition of their employment, is under threat – when there is a discrepancy between the amount of job security they would prefer and the amount that they actually have (Hartley et al, 1991). The notion of job insecurity thus entails a subjective element, although the reality of threatened or actual job loss can be very real. Job insecurity can be externally assigned (for example, by researchers) or can be self-reported by an individual.

Studies of job insecurity and its impact on health are most often cross-sectional and thus limited in their ability to establish causal associations with health outcomes. These and a few cohort studies report an association between perceived or attributed job insecurity and self-reported morbidity or psychological morbidity. However, little research has investigated the effect of job insecurity on mortality (except for studies that use unemployment as measure of job insecurity). Thus, the associations could be explained by elevated self-reporting of morbidities among those who self-report greater job insecurity.

The National Statistics Socioeconomic Classification (see **2.23 NS-SEC**) attempts to include some aspect of job security by including the size of organisation for which an individual works in its classification methodology.

Discussion point

Job insecurity has spread throughout the 1990s, particularly amongst professional workers.... The fear of redundancy is not the only aspect of job insecurity. Although many employees are not unduly worried about losing their jobs per se, they are extremely worried about the loss of valued job features, such as their status within the organisation and their opportunity for promotion ... the root cause of job insecurity and work intensification lies with the reduced staffing levels pursued by senior managers in response to the market pressures from their competitors and dominant stakeholders. (Burchell et al, 1999)

References

Burchell, B.J., Day, D., Hudson, M. et al (1999) 'Job insecurity and work intensification: flexibility and the changing boundaries of work', *Findings* 849, York: Joseph Rowntree Foundation.

Hartley, J., Jacobsson, D., Klandermans, P. and van Vuuren, T. (1991) *Job insecurity: Coping with jobs at risk*, London: Sage Publications.

Further reading

Bartley, M. and Ferrie, J. (2001) 'Glossary: unemployment, job insecurity, and health', *Journal of Epidemiology and Community Health*, vol 55, no 11, pp 776-81.

Ferrie, J. (2000) 'Is job insecurity harmful to health?', *Journal of the Royal Society of Medicine*, vol 94, pp 71-6.

See also: 2.25 Occupation-based measures; 2.31 Unemployment

2.23 National Statistics Socioeconomic Classification (NS-SEC)

From 2000 the UK National Statistics Socioeconomic Classification (NS-SEC) has replaced the Registrar General's Social Classes (RGSC). Details on the history, process and conversion between these schemes can be found on the National Statistics website (www.statistics.gov.uk). The NS-SEC is now used in the UK census, and all official statistics and surveys in the UK. While the RGSC measure is based simply on occupation (job title), NS-SEC is more complex and uses several pieces of information about somebody's job to classify their socioeconomic position.

The NS-SEC is explicitly based on differences between employment conditions and relations, similar to the Erikson and Goldthorpe class schema. People are placed in groups according to occupations with different employment relations and conditions, such as whether they have a wage rather than a salary, their prospects for promotion, job security, and levels of autonomy. The direct interpretation of associations between NS-SEC and health outcomes relies on the effect that conditions and relations of employment have on health; differences in material resources will also exist between the groups. Similar to the Erikson and Goldthorpe class schema, the NS-SEC is not a hierarchical classification, except for the grouping that collapses into three categories, which may be assumed to involve some kind of hierarchy.

Technical detail – National Statistics Socioeconomic Classification (NS-SEC)

NS-SEC (8 classes)		NS-SEC (5 classes)		NS-SEC (3 classes)	
I	Higher managerial and professional occupations	I	Managerial and professional occupations	I	Managerial and professional occupations
1.1	Large employers and higher managerial occupations				
1.2	Higher professional occupations				
2	Lower managerial and professional occupations				
3	Intermediate occupations	2	Intermediate occupations	2	Intermediate occupations
4	Small employers and own account workers	3	Small employers and own account workers		
5	Lower supervisory and technical occupations	4	Lower supervisory and technical occupations	3	Routine and manual occupations
6	Semi-routine occupations	5	Semi-routine and routine occupations		
7	Routine occupations				
8	Never worked and long-term unemployed		Never worked and long-term unemployed		Never worked and long-term unemployed

Example

Age-standardised rates of long-term illness or disability that restricts daily activities: by NS-SEC, April 2001, England and Wales

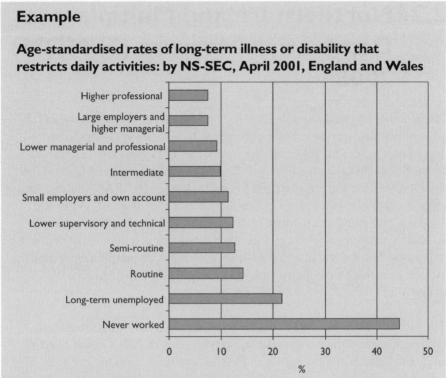

Source: Census, April 2001, Office for National Statistics (www.statistics.gov.uk/cci/nugget.asp?id=916)

Further reading

Chandola, T. (2000) 'Social class differences in mortality using the new UK National Statistics Socio-Economic Classification', *Social Science and Medicine*, vol 50, no 5, pp 641-9.

Drever, F., Doran, T. and Whitehead, M. (2004) 'Exploring the relation between class, gender, and self rated general health using the new socioeconomic classification. A study using data from the 2001 census', *Journal of Epidemiology and Community Health*, vol 58, pp 590-6.

Rose, D. and O'Reilly, K. (eds) (1997) *Constructing classes: Towards a new social classification for the UK*, Swindon: ESRC/ONS.

Weblinks

UK National Statistics NS-SEC:

www.statistics.gov.uk/methods_quality/ns_sec/default.asp

See also: 2.10 Erikson and Goldthorpe class schema; 2.25 Occupation-based measures; 2.26 Occupational social class – Registrar General's Social Classes (RGSC)

2.24 Northern Ireland Multiple Deprivation Measure (NIMDM) 2005

The Northern Ireland Multiple Deprivation Measure (NIMDM) is the official government deprivation index for Northern Ireland. As with government deprivation indices for other UK countries, the 2005 version was created by the Social Disadvantage Research Centre at the University of Oxford for the Northern Ireland Statistics and Research Agency (NISRA). The measure follows a similar methodology and format to those for England, Wales and Scotland, consisting of a number of deprivation 'domains' such as income, education and proximity to services, each consisting of a number of deprivation indicators. The domain scores have their own merit as specific deprivation indices, but are also combined to form a composite overall measure of deprivation.

The NIMDM 2005 was calculated for small areas across Northern Ireland known as super output areas (SOAs), aggregations of 2001 Census output areas similar to SOAs in England and Wales, and data zones in Scotland.

Technical detail
The domains and indicators in the NIMDM 2005 are as follows (extracted from NISRA, 2005).

Income deprivation
The purpose of this domain is to capture the proportions of the population experiencing income deprivation in an area.

Adults and children in Income Support households (includes lone parents and Minimum Income Guarantee recipients) (DSD) 2003

Adults and children in Income-based Jobseeker's Allowance households (DSD) 2003

Adults and children in Working Families Tax Credit households whose equivalised income (excluding Housing Benefit) is below 60% of median before housing costs (Inland Revenue and DSD) 2003

Adults and children in Disabled Person's Tax Credit households whose equivalised income (excluding Housing Benefits) is below 60% of median before housing costs (Inland Revenue and DSD) 2003

Employment deprivation

This domain measures employment deprivation conceptualised as involuntary exclusion of the working-age population from the world of work.

Unemployment claimant count (JUVOS) of women aged 18-59 and men aged 18-64 averaged over four quarters (DETI) 2003

Incapacity Benefit claimants women aged 18-59 and men aged 18-64 (DSD) 2003

Severe Disablement Allowance claimants women aged 18-59 and men aged 18-64 (DSD) 2003

Participants in New Deal for Young People (18-24 years) who are not included in the claimant count (DEL) 2003

Participants in New Deal for 25+ who are not included in the claimant count (DEL) 2003

Invalid Care Allowance claimants women aged 18-59 and men aged 18-64 (DSD) 2003

Health deprivation and disability

This domain identifies areas with relatively high rates of people who die prematurely or whose quality of life is impaired by poor health or who are disabled, across the whole population.

Years of potential life lost (Mortality data, NISRA) 1999-2003

Comparative illness and disability ratio (IS, AA, DLA, SDA, IB from DSD) 2003

A combined measure of two indicators: (i) individuals suffering from mood or anxiety disorders, based on prescribing (CSA) 2003 and (ii) suicides (NISRA) 1999-2003

People registered as having cancer (excluding non-melanoma skin cancers) (Northern Ireland Cancer Registry) 1999-2002

Education, skills and training deprivation

The purpose of the domain is to capture the extent of deprivation in education, skills and training in a local area.

Subdomain: Children/young people
GCSE/GNVQ points score (School Leavers Survey, DE) 1999/2000–2001/02
Key Stage 3 data (DE) 2002/03. Note: Key Stage 3 assessment is based on formal tests taken by pupils at the end of Key Stage 3 (approximately age 14) in English (and Irish – in Irish medium schools/units), Mathematics and Science
Proportions of those leaving school aged 16 and not entering further education (School Leavers Survey, DE) 1999/2000–2001/02
Absenteeism at secondary level (all absences) (SAER, DE) 2001/02 and 2002/03
Proportions of 17- to 20-year-olds who have not successfully applied for higher education (UCAS and DEL) 1999/2000–2002/03
Proportions of Year 11 and Year 12 pupils not in a grammar school (School Census, DE) 2003
Proportions of post-primary pupils with special educational needs in mainstream schools (School Census, DE) 2002/03

Subdomain: Working-age adults
Proportions of working-age adults (aged 25-59) in the area with no or low levels of qualification (NISRA) 2001

Proximity to services deprivation
The purpose of this domain is to measure the extent to which people have poor geographical access to certain key services, measured in terms of road distance to the nearest services.

Road distance to a GP premises (CSA) 2004
Road distance to an Accident and Emergency hospital (DHSSPS) 2004
Road distance to a dentist (CSA) 2004
Road distance to an optician (CSA) 2004
Road distance to a pharmacist (CSA) 2004
Road distance to a job centre or jobs and benefit office (DEL) 2004
Road distance to a post office (Post Office Ltd) 2004
Road distance to a food shop (Census of Employment) 2003
Road distance to the centre of a settlement of 10,000 or more people (NISRA) 2004

Living environment
The purpose of this domain is to identify deprivation relating to the environment in which people live.

Subdomain: Housing quality
SOA level housing stress (SDRC and NIHE, modelled NIHCS) 2001
Houses without central heating (NISRA) 2001

Subdomain: Housing access
Household overcrowding (NISRA) 2001 Census
LGD level rate of acceptances under the homelessness provisions of the Housing (Northern Ireland) Order 1988 and the Housing (Northern Ireland) Order 2003, assigned to the constituent SOAs (NIHE) 2003

Subdomain: Outdoor physical environment
SOA level local area problem score (SDRC and NIHE, modelled NIHCS) 2001

Crime and disorder
This domain measures the rate of crime and disorder at small area level.

Subdomain: Crime
Violence, robbery and public order (PSNI) April 2002-March 2004
Burglary (PSNI) April 2002-March 2004
Vehicle theft (PSNI) April 2002-March 2004
Criminal damage (PSNI) April 2002-March 2004

Subdomain: Disorder
Malicious and deliberate primary fires (NIFB) April 2002-March 2004
Disturbances (PSNI) April 2002-March 2004

References
NISRA (Northern Ireland Statistics and Research Agency) (2005) *The Northern Ireland Multiple Deprivation Measure 2005: Final report* (www.nisra.gov.uk).

See also: 2.8 Deprivation indices; 2.19 and 2.20 Indices of Deprivation 2000 and 2004; 2.29 Scottish Index of Multiple Deprivation (SIMD) 2006; 2.32 Welsh Index of Multiple Deprivation (WIMD) 2005

2.25 Occupation-based measures

Indicators based on occupation are widely used as measurements of socioeconomic position (SEP) (Hauser and Warren, 1997; Galobardes et al, 2006), particularly in the UK, where social stratification has traditionally been conceptualised in terms of someone's occupation. Although a range of indicators have been based on this occupational variable, they can have different theoretical bases and therefore a variety of interpretations. They usually represent Weber's notion of SEP as a reflection of an individual's place in society related to their social standing, income and education; characterise working relations between employers and employees; or, less frequently, characterise social class following Marx's principles of class relations and exploitation. In addition to measuring SEP, occupation can also be used as a proxy indicator for occupational exposures. This different use overlaps with SEP only due to the fact that most occupational exposures carrying a risk for health tend to occur among groups of lower SEP.

The current or longest held occupation of an individual is most frequently used to characterise adult SEP. However, with increasing interest in the role of SEP across the life course, some studies use occupations at different stages of adult life, in addition to parental occupation (as an indicator of childhood SEP), to capture SEP from across the life course. Social class at different times of the life course is also used to assess social mobility and its effects on health and other outcomes.

Strengths

The occupation of individuals is relatively easy to measure and is often available in routine data sources. Among some populations there may be less stigmatisation or embarrassment attached to reporting occupation than there is associated with other measures of SEP based on income or wealth and therefore the response to questions about occupation and the accuracy with which they are answered may be better.

Occupational measures are in some sense transferable: measures from one individual, or combinations of several individuals, can be used to characterise the SEP of others connected to them. For example, the occupation of the 'head of the household', or the 'highest status occupation in the household', can be used as an indicator of the SEP of dependants (such as children) or the household as a unit.

Limitations

Many occupational classification schemes have not been recently updated (details as to when they were first derived and whether they have been updated or not are given in entries for specific measures), and probably cannot account for today's occupational structure. The decrease in the number of people working in manual occupations, for example, with a concomitant increase in low-level service occupations has altered the stratification that occupation generates in terms of SEP. Classifications such as manual and non-manual worker may therefore lose some of their meaning in economies that include a large number of low-paid non-manual service jobs. This will result in cohort effects (that is, effects specific to groups born at the same time, but that differ between groups born at different times; see **4.1 Age-period cohort analysis (or effects)**) that should be taken into account to correctly interpret these associations. In addition, women have moved into the labour force in increasing numbers in recent decades, and occupational classification schemes based on male employment and stratification may well not be transferable to the work that women do. Using a husband's occupation to define a woman's SEP may have been appropriate for older generations but is unlikely to be the case for younger generations.

Another limitation shared by most occupation-based schemes is the fact that these indicators cannot be readily assigned to individuals who are not currently employed. Excluding this segment of the population may under-estimate socioeconomic differentials (Martikainen and Valkonen, 1999). Groups commonly excluded are retired individuals, people whose work is inside the home (most commonly women), the unemployed, students and people working in unpaid, informal or illegal jobs. Although previous occupation can be assigned to those who are retired and to some unemployed people, and husband's occupation is often used to assign women's SEP, this may inadequately index current circumstances.

Relatively recent occupation-based classification schemes, such as the National Statistics Socioeconomic Classification (NS-SEC), utilise a number of facets of employment (such as company size and supervisory responsibilities) rather than simply using 'occupation' (job title). This more sophisticated approach to occupational SEP classification begins to address these limitations to some extent, although it does not overcome them entirely.

Example

Occupation and health

Although occupational classifications measure particular aspects of SEP, they also share some more generic mechanisms that may explain the association between occupation and health-related outcomes. For example, occupation (parental or own adult) is strongly related to income and therefore any association between occupation-based SEP and health may indicate a direct relationship between material resources and health. Occupations reflect social standing or status and may be related to health outcomes because of certain privileges – such as easier access to better healthcare, access to education and more salubrious residential facilities – that are more easily achieved for those of higher standing. Occupation-based SEP may reflect social networks and psychosocial processes. Finally, as mentioned above, occupation-based SEP may be a proxy for occupational exposures and reflect specific toxic environmental or work task exposures with particular physical demands.

References

Galobardes, B., Shaw, M., Lawlor, D.A., Davey Smith, G. and Lynch J. (2006) 'Indicators of socioeconomic position', in M. Oakes, J. Kaufman and J. Jossey-Bass (eds) *Methods in social epidemiology*, London: John Wiley & Sons, Inc.

Hauser, R.M. and Warren, J.R. (1997) 'Socioeconomic indexes for occupations: a review, update, and critique', *Sociological Methodology*, vol 27, pp 177-298.

Martikainen, P. and Valkonen, T. (1999) 'Bias related to the exclusion of the economically inactive in studies on social class differences in mortality', *International Journal of Epidemiology*, vol 28, pp 899-904.

Further reading

Crompton, R. (1998) *Class and stratification: An introduction to current debates*, Cambridge: Polity Press.

Grint, K. (2000) *Work and society: A reader*, Cambridge: Polity Press.

Grint, K. (2005) *The sociology of work*, Cambridge: Polity Press.

See also: 1.7 Life course socioeconomic position; 1.14 Social class; 2.4 Cambridge Social Interaction and Stratification Scale (CAMSIS); 2.10 Erikson and Goldthorpe class schema; 2.23 National Statistics Socioeconomic Classification (NS-SEC); 2.26 Occupational social class – Registrar General's Social Classes (RGSC)

2.26 Occupational social class – Registrar General's Social Classes (RGSC)

The Registrar General's Annual Report using data from the 1911 Census presented a summary of occupations representing 'social grades' separately from an industrial classification. It was the official classification in Britain until 2000, and it was known, prior to 1990, as the Registrar General's Social Classes (RGSC).

This scale was based on the prestige or social standing that a given occupation has in society. After revisions in 1990 this measure was more explicitly related to the skills needed to perform a particular occupation. It is widely used in Britain and in other European countries. As (theoretically) a measure of prestige or social standing, association with health outcomes should be interpreted as due to the advantages provided by increased prestige. In practice it is often interpreted as an indicator of both social standing and material reward and resources.

Occupations are categorised into six levels or classes that can also be reduced to two broad categories of manual and non-manual occupations; a seventh category includes all individuals in the armed forces irrespective of their rank therein, which is generally excluded in health studies.

Technical detail – The Registrar General's Social Classes		
I	Professional	Non-manual
II	Intermediate	
III-N	Skilled non-manual	
III-M	Skilled manual	Manual
IV	Partly skilled	
V	Unskilled	
VI	Armed forces	

Strengths

A key strength of this measure is its past official status in Britain, and hence its widespread use in vital statistics, population censuses and surveys over a long time period. Many European countries have created adaptations of this classification, which makes results from these international studies more comparable.

Limitations

This classification has been criticised for its weak theoretical basis given the subjectivity by which the prestige associated with a particular occupation is assigned. In addition, recent changes in the occupational structure, such as the increase in service jobs and the decrease in unskilled and semi-skilled manual occupations, and the increasing number of women in the labour market, have not been incorporated, and whether it classifies today's jobs structure is questionable. Based on these criticisms, the Office for National Statistics (ONS) in the UK has since 2000 used the new UK National Statistics Socioeconomic Classification (NS-SEC) as its official occupation classification.

The Registrar General's classification does not include people without occupation, who remain unclassified, a group that generally is of lower socioeconomic position (SEP), but varies depending on the occupation-based classification being used.

Example
Age-adjusted 21-year all-cause and cardiovascular disease (CVD) death rates (per 10,000 person years) in the Collaborative Study, UK

	All cause		CVD	
	n deaths	Death rate	n deaths	Death rate
I	156	101.1	65	48.0
II	242	110.0	138	66.8
IIIN	293	139.5	155	79.8
IIIM	530	153.0	273	86.4
IV	334	152.6	172	87.7
V	84	170.5	38	78.7
Trend	$p=0.0001$		$p=0.0001$	

Source: Davey Smith et al (1998)

In this example, all-cause and CVD mortality rates increase with decreasing social class.

References

Davey Smith, G., Hart, C., Hole, D., MacKinnon, P., Gillis, C., Watt, G., Blane, D. and Hawthorne, V. (1998) 'Education and occupational social class: which is the more important indicator of mortality risk?', *Journal of Epidemiology and Community Health*, vol 52, pp 153-60.

Further reading

Leete, R. and Fox, J. (1977) 'Registrar General's social classes: origins and uses', *Population Trends*, vol 8, pp 1-7.

Rose, M. (2005) *Official social classifications in the UK*, Social Research Update 9, University of Surrey (www.soc.surrey.ac.uk/sru/SRU9.html).

See also: 2.10 Erikson and Goldthorpe class schema; 2.23 National Statistics Socioeconomic Classification (NS-SEC); 2.25 Occupation-based measures

2.27 Overcrowding

The extent to which people live in overcrowded housing is commonly used as an indicator of socioeconomic position (SEP). Together with other indicators of sanitary conditions, such as access to clean water and the presence of damp and mould, overcrowding gained much attention from the public health movement of the 19th and early 20th centuries (Shaw, 2004).

Overcrowding is essentially a measure of population density at the household, or micro, level. It is usually indicated by the ratio of the number of residents to the number of rooms in a dwelling, although the concept of sufficiency is sometimes preferred (see Example box); sometimes the number of people per dwelling is used. It is assumed that a high level of overcrowding will correspond with, or indicate, a lower general SEP. Those with greater resources will usually use those resources to improve their living conditions and this includes, but is not limited to, acquiring a more spacious home.

Example

Sufficiency
The *Canadian National Occupancy Standard* is a measure of sufficiency of rooms according to household size and characteristics. It assesses the bedroom requirements of a household by specifying that: there should be no more than two people per bedroom; children younger than five years of age of different sexes may reasonably share a bedroom; children five years of age or older of opposite sex should have separate bedrooms; children younger than 18 years of age and of the same sex may reasonably share a bedroom; and single household members 18 years or older should have a separate bedroom, as should parents or couples (Booth and Carroll, 2005).

Overcrowding can affect health in a number of ways. In a direct, physical sense, overcrowding can be related to the more rapid transmission of airborne infectious diseases. For example, severe overcrowding has been related to the prevalence of tuberculosis (Acevedo-Garcia, 2000). The sharing of cooking and washing facilities and the close proximity of daily living may also lead to a greater likelihood of diarrhoea.

Overcrowding may also have a detrimental effect on mental health, although there is less convincing evidence here (OPDM, 2004). It has been argued that living in overcrowded conditions can lead to psychological distress, leading to anxiety and depression (and potentially to aggression and violence). However, it must also be taken into consideration that social isolation and living alone – living with too few people rather than too many – can have detrimental effects on health. A study of women in London found a J-shaped relationship between household density and psychological symptoms (Gabe and Williams, 1993), a relationship that persisted when controlling for other socioeconomic variables. As psychosocial aspects of health and well-being receive greater research attention, this and other aspects of housing conditions and the quality of the home environment may be more closely investigated.

Overcrowding has most frequently been used as a component of area-based deprivation indicators (with other measures such as not having sole access to a bathroom or kitchen) including the Townsend and Carstairs Indices. For example, the Townsend Index of Deprivation includes overcrowding and non-owner-occupation (as well as unemployment and lack of access to a car). Such composite indicators have been found to correlate strongly with measures of health and premature mortality at the ecological level (Benach et al, 2003).

Strengths

An advantage of this indicator is that it can be easily calculated once data on the number of rooms and number of residents have been collected (sufficiency requires further information on the type of rooms, and sometimes ages and relationships of household members). These component data are traditionally collected in population censuses (see Technical detail below), and overcrowding is thus useful because it is available for the whole population, albeit at 10-year intervals.

Limitations

This measure is fairly crude in that it includes the number of rooms, but not their size or quality. Overcrowding is usually treated as a dichotomous rather than a continuous variable, which implies that the cut-off point is meaningful rather than arbitrary.

Changes to the cut-off point, and what counts as a 'room', can lead to difficulty with comparisons at different time points.

Other indicators of housing may have more currency in terms of relating to SEP. For instance, in the UK the location of a house near to a particular school, rather than its size and the extent of overcrowding, may be a better indicator of the SEP of the household – people may be sacrificing number of rooms in the short term for the long-term prospects for the life course SEP of their children.

Technical detail – Overcrowding and the 2001 Census

In 2001 the Census asked:

How many rooms do you have for use only by your household?

- *Do not count* bathrooms, toilets, halls or landings, or rooms that can only be used for storage such as cupboards.
- *Do count* all other rooms, for example kitchens, living rooms, bedrooms, utility rooms and studies.

If two rooms have been converted into one, count them as one room.

There were 24.5 million households recorded in the UK at the 2001 Census. Just under half a million (1.9%) had more people than rooms. About one million households – 4.3% – had one or two people living in eight or more rooms.

Source: Wheeler et al (2005)

References

Acevedo-Garcia, D. (2000) 'Residential segregation and the epidemiology of infectious diseases', *Social Science & Medicine*, vol 51, pp 1143-61.

Benach, J., Yasui, Y., Borrell, C., Pasarin, M., Martinez, J. and Daponte, A. (2003) 'The public health burden of material deprivation: excess mortality in leading causes of death in Spain', *Preventive Medicine*, vol 36, pp 300-8.

Booth, A. and Carroll, N. (2005) *Overcrowding and indigenous health in Australia*, Discussion paper no 498, Canberra: Centre for Economic Policy Research, Australian National University.

Gabe, J. and Williams, P. (1993) 'Women, crowding and mental health', in R. Burridge and D. Ormandy (eds) *Unhealthy housing: Research, remedies and reform*, New York, NY: Spon Press, pp 191-208.

ODPM (Office of the Deputy Prime Minister) (2004) *The impact of overcrowding on health and education: A review of the evidence and literature*, Housing Research Summary Number 210, London: ODPM.

Shaw, M. (2004) 'Housing and public health', *Annual Review of Public Health*, vol 25, pp 397-418.

Wheeler, B., Shaw, M., Mitchell, R. and Dorling, D. (2005) *Life in Britain: Using millennial Census data to understand poverty, inequality and place*, Bristol: The Policy Press (www. shef.ac.uk/sasi/research/life_in_britain.htm) [A pack of 10 reports, a technical, summary and five posters produced for the Joseph Rowntree Foundation].

See also: 2.1 Amenities; 2.6 Carstairs Deprivation Index; 2.8 Deprivation indices; 2.12 Housing conditions; 2.30 Townsend Index of Deprivation

2.28 Poverty – the official government measure

The concept of poverty has been operationalised into something that can be measured in numerous ways. A traditional approach to measuring poverty is to use a low-income threshold below which an individual or household is deemed to be living in poverty (see **3.4 Households Below Average Income (HBAI)**). An alternative method is to use a consensual measure of poverty that involves asking people about their standard of living and the specific items that they consider people need to have in order not to be considered to be living in poverty (see **2.3 Breadline Britain and the Millennium Survey of Poverty and Social Exclusion**).

The current official governmental view on poverty is that it is a multidimensional issue and not limited to low income (Townsend and Kennedy, 2004). Therefore a range of indicators has been used to monitor poverty and these are reported in an annual series of reports called *Opportunity for all*. There are separate indicators for children and young people, people of working age and older people, and there is also a set of indicators for communities (see box below).

Many of these indicators are not actually measures of poverty, but indicators of health, crime, educational attainment and factors that are often related to poverty.

Opportunity for all **poverty indicators for children and young people**
Children in workless households
Low income (relative, absolute and persistent measures)
Teenage pregnancy (teenage conceptions, and teenage parents not in education, employment and training)
Key Stage 1 attainment (7-year-olds) in Sure Start areas
Key Stage 2 attainment (11-year-olds)
16-year-olds with at least one GCSE
19-year-olds with at least a Level 2 qualification
Truancies
School exclusions
Educational attainment of children looked after by local authorities
16- to 18-year-olds in learning

Infant mortality

Serious unintentional injury

Smoking rates (for pregnant women, and children aged 11-15)

Re-registrations on Child Protection Register

Housing that falls below the set standard of decency

Opportunity for all poverty indicators for people of working age

Employment rate

Employment rates of disadvantaged groups: people with disabilities; lone
   parents; minority ethnic people; older workers, lowest qualified

Working-age people in workless households

Working-age people without a qualification at NVQ Level 2 or higher

Long periods on income-related benefits

Low income (relative, absolute and persistent measures)

Smoking rates: all adults; manual socioeconomic groups

Death rates from suicide and undetermined injury

Rough sleepers

Use of Class A drugs

Opportunity for all poverty indicators for older people

Low income (relative, absolute and persistent measures)

People contributing to a non-state pension

Amount contributed to a non-state pension

People making continuous contributions to non-state pensions

Healthy life expectancy at age 65

Being helped to live independently: receiving intensive home care; receiving
   any community-based care

Housing that falls below the set standard of decency

Fear of crime

Opportunity for all poverty indicators for communities

Employment rates in deprived areas

Rate of domestic burglary

Housing that falls below the set standard of decency

Households in fuel poverty

Life expectancy at birth

Attainment gap at Key Stage 2 (11-year-olds)

Road accident casualties in deprived areas

For individual indicator summaries see
ww.dwp.gov.uk/ofa/indicators/complete.asp

References

Townsend, I. and Kennedy, S. (2004) *Poverty: Measures and targets*, House of Commons Research Paper 04/23, London: House of Commons Library.

Further reading

Spicker, P. (2007) *The idea of poverty*, Bristol: The Policy Press.

Weblinks

Opportunity for all:
www.dwp.gov.uk/ofa

See also: 1.1 Deprivation; 1.10 Poverty; 2.3 Breadline Britain and the Millennium Survey of Poverty and Social Exclusion; 2.7 Child poverty – the official government measure; 2.16 Income; 3.4 Households Below Average Income (HBAI)

2.29 Scottish Index of Multiple Deprivation (SIMD) 2006

The Scottish Index of Multiple Deprivation (SIMD) 2006 is an update of the SIMD 2003 and 2004, using updated data and a recently introduced small area geography called 'data zones'. The SIMD produced by the Scottish Executive and based on work developed by the Social Disadvantage Research Centre at the University of Oxford, covers all of Scotland and can be used to identify area-level relative deprivation.

The SIMD 2006 is made up of seven domains and 37 indicators measuring both individual and area characteristics (see box below). Compared to the SIMD 2004 the SIMD 2006 includes changes to methodology, improvements to existing data sources, a new crime domain and a public transportation subdomain; the two are therefore not directly comparable. The principles behind its construction are based on the work of Townsend and others in defining and measuring poverty – deprivation is seen as a multidimensional concept where standards are defined in relation to social norms or expectations. It is thus a relative rather than absolute concept. The technical report (see weblinks below) includes details of transformations and weights applied to the data.

SIMD 2006: Domains

Current income
Number of adults (aged 15-59) claiming Income Support (DWP) April 2005
Number of adults (aged 60+) claiming Guaranteed Pension Credit (DWP) May 2005
Number of children (aged 0-15) dependent on a claimant of Income Support (DWP) April 2005
Number of adults claiming (all) Jobseeker's Allowance (DWP) April 2005
Number of children (aged 0-15) dependent on a claimant of Jobseeker's Allowance (all) (DWP) April 2005

Employment
Working age unemployment claimant count averaged over 12 months (NOMIS) 2005
Working age Incapacity Benefit claimants, men aged under 65 and women aged under 60 (DWP) August 2005

Working age Severe Disablement Allowance claimants (DWP) August 2005
Working age compulsory New Deal participants – New Deal for the
   under 25s and New Deal for the 25+ not included in the unemployment
   claimant count (DWP) August 2005

Health
Standardised Mortality Ratio (ISD) 2001-04
Hospital episodes related to alcohol use (ISD) 2001-04
Hospital episodes related to drug use (ISD) 2001-04
Comparative illness factor (DWP) 2005
Emergency admissions to hospital (ISD) 2001-04
Proportion of population being prescribed drugs for anxiety, depression or
   psychosis (ISD) 2004
Proportion of live singleton births of low birth weight (ISD) 2001-04

Education skills and training
School pupil absences (attendance returns) 2003/04-2004/05
Pupil performance on SQA at Stage 4 (SQA) 2002/03-2004/05
Working age people with no qualifications (Census) 2001
17 to 21-year-olds enrolling into higher education (HESA) 2002/03-2004/05
People aged 16-18 not in full-time education (DWP) 2005 (HESA) 2004/05

Geographic access
Subdomain: Drive time
Drive time to a GP (OS) 2005
Drive time to a petrol station (Catalist) 2006
Drive time to a post office (PointX) 2006
Drive time to shopping facilities (CACI) 2006
Drive time to a primary school (Scottish Executive) 2005
Drive time to a secondary school (Scottish Executive) 2005

Subdomain: Public transport
Public transport time to a GP (OS) 2005
Public transport time to a post office (PointX) 2005
Public transport time to shopping facilities (CACI) 2006

Housing
Persons in households that are overcrowded (Census) 2001
Persons in households without central heating (Census) 2001

Crime
Recorded crimes of violence (Scottish Police Forces) 2004
Recorded domestic housebreaking (Scottish Police Forces) 2004
Recorded vandalism (Scottish Police Forces) 2004
Recorded drugs offences (Scottish Police Forces) 2004
Recorded minor assault (Scottish Police Forces) 2004

Further reading

Bailey, N., Flint, J., Goodlad, R., Shucksmith, M., Fitzpatrick, S. and Pryce, G. (2003) *Measuring deprivation in Scotland: Developing a long-term strategy: Final report,* Edinburgh: Scottish Executive Central Statistics Unit (www.scotland.gov.uk/ Publications/2003/09/18197/26536).

Weblinks

www.scotland.gov.uk/topics/statistics/SIMD/overview
www.scotland.gov.uk/topics/statistics/SIMD/background-data-2006

See also: 1.1 Deprivation; 1.10 Poverty; 2.8 Deprivation indices; 2.19 and 2.20 Indices of Deprivation 2000 and 2004

2.30 Townsend Index of Deprivation

The Townsend Index of Deprivation (also known as the Townsend Score or the Townsend Material Deprivation Score) is a measure of multiple deprivation for areas. It was developed by Professor Peter Townsend, who has been at the forefront of poverty studies since the 1950s. The Index, originally calculated using 1981 Census data, but which can also be derived from 1991 Census data, is based on four variables selected to be direct indicators of condition or state of deprivation:

- *Unemployment:* percentage of economically active residents aged 16-59/64 who are unemployed (representing lack of material resources and insecurity).
- *Car ownership:* percentage of private households who do not possess a car (a proxy indicator of income).
- *Home ownership:* percentage of private households not owner-occupied (a proxy indicator of wealth).
- *Overcrowding:* percentage of private households with more than one person per room (representing material living conditions).

The four variables that make up the Townsend Score are combined together in an overall deprivation score, with each variable being given an equal weight (the variables are first transformed to produce more normal distributions). The higher the score, the greater the deprivation in that area. The average is 0, and scores may be negative (less deprived) or positive (more deprived).

Strengths

The Townsend Index is probably the most widely used area-based measure of deprivation in studies of health; it has also been widely used by local authorities and councils for comparing the levels of deprivation across small areas. Until the introduction of the Index of Multiple Deprivation (IMD) in 2000 it was considered the best available indicator of material deprivation available. It can be calculated for the whole of the UK (the IMD only covers England, and similar indices for the other three countries of the UK are derived separately, making them incomparable) and for small areas (enumeration districts, wards).

Limitations

As each area is given a score, it can only be used to rank areas and to compare their levels of deprivation; the score itself has no value. It does not tell you what proportion of people in an area are deprived. Because it includes car ownership, it is a better indicator of urban than rural deprivation. Changes in the score for an area between 1981 and 1991 cannot be taken as indicative of reducing or increasing relative deprivation, primarily because of changes in the proportions and social characteristics of car and home ownership. As the Index uses census data, it can only be derived every 10 years. The 2001 Census changed the way that the number of rooms were counted, which affects the overcrowding element of this indicator, and hence there is ongoing discussion among analysts as to whether the Townsend Score should be calculated from 2001 Census data.

Further reading

Hoare, J. (2003) 'Comparison of area-based inequality measures and disease morbidity in England, 1994-1998', *Health Statistics Quarterly*, vol 18, pp 18-24.

Townsend, P., Phillimore, P. and Beattie, A. (1988) *Health and deprivation: Inequality and the North*, London: Croom Helm.

See also: 1.1 Deprivation; 1.10 Poverty; 2.6 Carstairs Deprivation Index; 2.8 Deprivation indices

2.31 Unemployment

While the common definition of unemployment – not being in paid work – is fairly straightforward, official definitions of unemployment can vary greatly over time and in different countries. These official definitions determine who is entitled to financial support (which can be of different forms; see Bartley and Ferrie, 2001). Usually, 'unemployed' refers to someone of working age (older than the minimum age requirement and younger than retirement age) who does not have a job and/or is actively seeking a job. Thus, unemployed people are excluded from the workforce, although they are part of the working-age population (that is, they are in the age range considered to be eligible for work). Long-term unemployment is usually considered to be when a person is unemployed for a year or longer.

While unemployment is a feature of individuals, unemployment *rates* are features of societies or areas within that society. The unemployment rate of an area is seen as an indicator of economic success or failure and has often been used in indices of deprivation, due to the association of unemployment with low income and poverty.

Discussion point

On the publication of a report on nutrition and health by the British Medical Association in 1933:

> Their report produced no little uneasiness when it was found that the diet which they estimated as the minimum necessary for existence was such that the mass of the unemployed ... especially those in the Distressed Areas, had an income which prevented them from obtaining it.

> ... the poor unemployed worker looked on at this new capitalist game of treating human beings like so many test-tubes. There was much talk of calories, alphabetical vitamins, proteins, carbohydrates, fats, and grammes, which all sounded like a foreign language to the ordinary unemployed worker whose family was having to exist on a diet composed chiefly of potatoes, bread, margarine, tea, and condensed milk. (Hannington, 1937)

Unemployment does not occur at random. People working in manual and unskilled occupations, in occupations that are not well paid and that involve hazardous exposures, are more likely to experience unemployment. Moreover, independently of individual characteristics, the chances of someone being unemployed are highly dependent on a country's overall economic situation and that of their immediate geographical area. Interventions to reduce unemployment that tackle only individual characteristics, for example, through retraining, are unlikely to have a great impact in reducing the proportion of unemployed people when overall unemployment rates are high.

Discussion point

After the steel strike came the year of the giro. Unemployment roared to two million, chased towards three million, and Norman Tebbitt famously said the unemployed should get on their bikes and look for work. Unemployment was the result of the unemployed not trying hard enough. In which case what a peculiar economic century we had.

The population must have gone through a period of laziness at the end of the 19th century, then felt a sudden spurt of energy and got jobs. Until the 1930s, when they got lazy again. Then they perked up around 1938, which was handy as it was just in time for the war. This was fine until 1980, when everyone changed their mind and decided to stay in bed all day, which makes sense as this coincides with the invention of the duvet. (Steel, 2001, p 81)

Strengths

Using unemployment as a measure of socioeconomic position (SEP) has the advantage that it is fairly straightforward to measure. However, it may also be useful to know the duration of unemployment, as sustained periods of being unemployed will have very different financial and health implications compared to brief periods of unemployment cushioned by redundancy payments.

Limitations

Many studies have reported an association between employment status and health such that unemployed people have worse health outcomes in terms of self-reported health (see Example below), poorer mental health and also excess mortality (Bartley et al, 2006). However, the results of cross-sectional studies may be due to health selection, that is, people with worse health are more likely to be unemployed in the first place, rather than to become ill due to the effects of unemployment. Therefore, the effect of unemployment on health is best studied through longitudinal studies, which can confirm that illness followed, rather than preceded, unemployment. However, in such studies it is also important to evaluate the extent to which poor health contributes to the chances of unemployment, as this is likely to constitute a cycle that is difficult to break.

Example

Work insecurity and self-reported general health at age 23 (National Child Development Study)

Previous spells of unemployment	Self-reported general health	
	Excellent/good (*n*=4,090)	Fair/poor (*n*=336)
0	94%	6%
1	92%	8%
2+	84%	16%

Source: Blane et al (1996)

References

Bartley, M. and Ferrie, J. (2001) 'Glossary: unemployment, job insecurity, and health', *Journal of Epidemiology and Community Health*, vol 55, no 11, pp 776-81.

Bartley, M., Ferrie, J. and Montgomery, S. (2006) 'Health and the labour market: unemployment, non-employment, and job insecurity', in M. Marmot and R. Wilkinson (eds) *Social determinants of health* (2nd edn), Oxford: Oxford University Press.

Blane, D., Brunner, E. and Wilkinson, R. (eds) (1996) *Health and social organization: Towards a health policy for the twenty-first century*, London: Routledge.

Hannington, W. (1937) *The problem of distressed areas*, reprinted in G. Davey Smith, D. Dorling and M. Shaw (eds) (2001) *Poverty, inequality and health in Britain: 1800-2000: A reader*, Bristol: The Policy Press, pp 198-9.

Steel, M. (2001) *Reasons to be cheerful*, New York, NY: Simon & Schuster.

See also: 2.8 Deprivation indices; 2.22 Job insecurity

2.32 Welsh Index of Multiple Deprivation (WIMD) 2005

The Welsh Index of Multiple Deprivation (WIMD) 2005 is the official measure of small area deprivation for Wales. It was updated from, and replaces, the WIMD 2000. It is a measure of multiple deprivation at the small area level, based on the idea of distinct domains of deprivation that can be measured separately. The overall WIMD 2005 is conceptualised as a weighted area-level aggregation of these individual dimensions.

As with other deprivation indices, if area A ranks more highly than area B it is correct to say that area A is more deprived, but not that area B is more affluent (it is less deprived; the Index does not measure affluence or wealth). The WIMD cannot be directly compared to the other UK indices of deprivation, the Scottish Index of Multiple Deprivation (SIMD), the Indices of Deprivation (England) or the Northern Ireland Multiple Deprivation Measure. The domains of the WIMD 2005 are detailed here.

WIMD 2005: Domains

Income
Claimants, partners and children of Income Support claimants (DWP) August 2004
Claimants, partners and children of Income-based Jobseeker's Allowance claimants (DWP) August 2004
Claimants, partners and children of Working Families Tax Credit claimants (DWP/HM Revenue and Customs) August 2002
Claimants, partners and children of Disabled Person's Tax Credit claimants (DWP/HM Revenue and Customs) August 2002

Employment
Claimants of Incapacity Benefit – women aged under 60 and men aged under 65 (DWP) April 2004
Claimants of Severe Disablement Allowance – women aged under 60 and men aged under 65 (DWP) April 2004
Participants on options for New Deal for Young People and intensive activity period for New Deal 25 plus (DWP) June 2004

Health

Standardised limiting long-term illness (2001 Census)

Standardised mortality ratio for all causes of death for all ages
(National Public Health Service for Wales) 1999-2003

Cancer standardised incidence ratio (Welsh Cancer Intelligence and
Surveillance Unit) 1994-2004

Education, skills and training

Average point score at Key Stage 2 (National Curriculum Assessments,
Welsh Assembly Government) 2004

Average point score at Key Stage 3 (National Curriculum Assessments,
Welsh Assembly Government) 2004

Average point score at Key Stage 4 (Welsh Examination Database, Welsh
Assembly Government) 2004

Proportion of adults with low or no qualifications (2001 Census)

Proportion of 17- and 18-year-olds not entering further or higher
education (HM Revenue and Customs) 2004

Secondary school absence rates (Pupil Attendance Database, Welsh
Assembly Government) 2004

Housing

Households lacking central heating (2001 Census)

Household overcrowding, excluding all student households (2001 Census)

Physical environment

Air quality (Environment Agency Wales) 2005

Air emissions (Environment Agency Wales) 2005

Proportion of population living within 1km of a waste disposal site
(Environment Agency Wales) 2005

Proportion of population living within 1km of a significant industrial source
(Environment Agency Wales) 2005

Proportion of population living in an area with a significant risk of flooding
(Environment Agency Wales) 2005

Geographical access to services by bus and walking

Proportion of population within 10 minutes of a food shop by walking and
bus (Local Government Data Unit, Wales) 2005

Proportion of population within 15 minutes of a GP surgery by walking and
bus (Local Government Data Unit, Wales) 2005

Proportion of population within 15 minutes of a primary school by walking
and bus (Local Government Data Unit, Wales) 2005

Proportion of population within 30 minutes of a secondary school by walking and bus (Local Government Data Unit, Wales) 2005

Proportion of population within 30 minutes of an NHS dentist by walking and bus (Local Government Data Unit, Wales) 2005

Proportion of population within 15 minutes of a post office by walking and bus (Local Government Data Unit, Wales) 2005

Proportion of population within 15 minutes of a public library by walking and bus (Local Government Data Unit, Wales) 2005

Proportion of population within 20 minutes of a leisure centre or swimming pool by walking and bus (Local Government Data Unit, Wales) 2005

Weblinks

Information and guidance:

http://new.wales.gov.uk/topics/statistics/theme/wimd2005/?lang=en

Domains:

www.lgdu-wales.gov.uk/eng/Project.asp?id=SX9C17-A77FB4F3

See also: 1.1 Deprivation; 1.10 Poverty; 2.8 Deprivation indices; 2.19 and 2.20 Indices of Deprivation 2000 and 2004

Part Three
Measures of inequality

3.1 Absolute differences

Both absolute and relative differences are measures of inequality since they examine the absolute or relative difference in an outcome (for example, health or disease status) by categories of an exposure (for example, social class groups).

An absolute difference (also known as absolute effect) refers to the consequence of an exposure, expressed as the *difference* between proportions, means, rates, risk, etc, as opposed to being expressed as a *ratio* of these (see **3.9 Relative differences**). The exposure of interest, forming the categories we wish to compare, could be a measure of socioeconomic position (SEP), sex, ethnicity, age, geographical area, time period and so on.

Since the absolute difference depends on how common the outcome of interest is in the population under study it may vary even when the relative difference remains constant. For example, a relative risk of 2 for heart disease comparing the least affluent to the most affluent groups may occur if the risk of heart disease is 50 per 1,000 in the least affluent group and 25 per 1,000 in the most affluent group (absolute difference = 25 per 1,000) or if the risk is 5 per 1,000 in the least affluent group and 2.5 per 1,000 in the most affluent group (absolute difference = 2.5 per 1,000). It is also possible that over time, as the frequency of an outcome decreases, the absolute difference could decrease as the relative difference increases (Regidor, 2004).

Strengths

An absolute difference can provide a measure of the number of lives saved or diseases prevented if the experience in the 'worst' group were the same as that in the 'best' group (see Example below).

Limitations

There is much debate about whether inequalities should be expressed as absolute or relative differences (see, for example, Wagstaff et al, 1991; Mackenbach and Kunst, 1997; Ebrahim, 2002; Oliver et al, 2002; Low and Low, 2005; Shaw et al, 2005). Those arguing for one or the other method often do so after results have been obtained and to some extent their choice is determined by the particular message they want to express. Absolute and relative differences represent different aspects of the data and both are valid measurements. In epidemiology, relative risks are taken as better indices of aetiological (causal) effect, absolute differences as better indices of public health importance. Inequalities in health have relevance to both aetiology and public health and ideally both absolute and relative differences (or results that would allow both to be calculated) should be presented in research and reports of inequality.

Example

In the Independent Inquiry into Inequalities in Health in England (referred to as the 'Acheson Inquiry') all-cause mortality was presented for different social classes so that absolute and relative differences could be calculated. All-cause mortality in men aged 20-64 years in 1991-93 was 806 per 100,000 for those in social class V and 280 per 100,000 for those in social class I. The difference in mortality (absolute difference) is 806 per 100,000 minus 280 per 100,000, which equals 526 per 100,000. Thus for every 100,000 men in social class V, 526 deaths would be delayed or prevented if men in this social class had the same health experience as those in social class I. This compares to a relative risk (*relative difference*) of 2.88 (806/280).

Note: Social class here refers to the UK Registrar General's classification of occupational social classes (see **2.26**). Note also that the comparison between the two extreme groups of social class is sometimes referred to as the *range* of inequality.

Source: Acheson (1998)

References

Acheson, Sir Donald (1998) *Independent Inquiry into Inequalities in Health*, London: The Stationery Office.

Ebrahim, S. (2002) 'Addressing health inequalities', *Lancet*, vol 360, p 1691.

Low, A. and Low, A. (2005) 'Health inequalities under New Labour: relative rather than absolute gaps are more important over time and place', *BMJ*, vol 330, p 1507.

Mackenbach, J.P. and Kunst, A.E. (1997) 'Measuring the magnitude of socio-economic inequalities in health: an overview of available measures illustrated with two examples from Europe', *Social Science & Medicine*, vol 44, pp 757-71.

Oliver, A., Healey, A. and Le Grand, J. (2002) 'Addressing health inequalities', *Lancet*, vol 360, pp 565-7.

Regidor, E. (2004) 'Measures of health inequalities: part 2', *Journal of Epidemiology and Community Health*, vol 58, pp 900-3.

Shaw, M., Davey Smith, G. and Dorling, D. (2005) 'Health inequalities under New Labour: authors' reply', *BMJ*, vol 330, pp 1507-8.

Wagstaff, A., Paci, P. and van Doorslaer, E. (1991) 'On the measurement of inequalities in health', *Social Science & Medicine*, vol 33, pp 545-57.

See also: 1.14 Social class; 3.7 Range; 3.9 Relative differences

3.2 Dissimilarity Index

The Dissimilarity Index was originally developed in demography as a measure of residential segregation (Duncan and Duncan, 1955). For example, in the context of economic segregation among neighbourhoods within a city, the Dissimilarity Index measures the proportion or number of low-income (or conversely high-income) people who would have to move to a different neighbourhood to achieve an economic distribution within each neighbourhood that was similar to that of the city as a whole. In this case, the Dissimilarity Index is a summary measure of the inequality between each neighbourhood's economic composition and the overall economic composition.

This idea can be extended to any quantity that is unevenly distributed within and across neighbourhoods, such as health. We can think of the Dissimilarity Index as a summary measure of the inequality between, for example, each social class's low birth weight (LBW) rate and the LBW rate of the whole population. In this case, the Dissimilarity Index would be interpreted as the number or proportion of LBW cases that would have to be redistributed across social class groups for each group's LBW rate to be the same as the rate in the whole population.

Technical detail

The formula for the *relative* Dissimilarity Index with respect to health is given by Wagstaff and colleagues (1991) as:

$$\frac{1}{2}\sum_{j=1}^{J}\left|s_{jh} - s_{ip}\right|$$

where j indexes social groups, s_{jh} is the jth group's share of health (for example, share of all LBW cases) and s_{ip} is the jth group's share of the total population. The *absolute* version of the Dissimilarity Index is calculated by multiplying the relative Dissimilarity Index by the total number of cases to determine the absolute number of cases that need to be redistributed across groups.

Strengths

The Dissimilarity Index can be easily calculated, and can be expressed in absolute and relative terms.

Limitations

The Dissimilarity Index is insensitive to the direction of inequality. It is only sensitive to uneven distribution across social groups. Over time, if inequality were unevenly distributed such that more disease was concentrated among the poor and at a subsequent time the distribution had reversed and was then equally concentrated among the rich, the Dissimilarity Index would not change. It is arguable that a 'good' measure of inequality should be sensitive to which social groups bear the uneven burden of disease. Are we more concerned when excess disease occurs among the poor or the rich? If so, our inequality measure should register this as it changes over time, and the Dissimilarity Index is not recommended for measuring inequality for that reason.

Example

The table below shows how one might calculate the absolute and relative Dissimilarity Index for a hypothetical health outcome. A comparison of columns (3) and (5) shows that the share of cases is lower than the share in the total population for all groups except C, who represent 13.9% of all cases but only 10.5% of the population. Similarly for the absolute Dissimilarity Index, a comparison of columns (2) and (6) shows that if all groups experienced the population rate, more cases would be observed for all groups except for C. The relative Dissimilarity Index in this case is 3.4, which means that 3.4% of the 17,186 cases need to be redistributed across social groups to eliminate the inequality. In absolute terms, this means redistributing 592 cases.

Social group	Rate	Cases	% of total cases	Population	% of total population	Cases if no inequality	Index relative	Index absolute
	(1)	(2)	(3)	(4)	(5)	(6)	|(3)−(5)|	|(2)−(6)|
A	5.7	133	0.8	2,316,609	1.3	226	0.5	93
B	8.7	1,648	9.6	18,850,492	10.7	1,835	1.1	187
C	12.9	2,395	13.9	18,518,113	10.5	1,803	3.4	592
D	9.5	13,010	75.7	136,864,686	77.5	13,323	1.8	313
Total	9.7	17,186	100.0	176,549,900	100.0	17,186	3.4%	592

References

Duncan, O. and Duncan, B. (1955) 'A methodological analysis of segregation indices', *American Sociological Review*, vol 20, pp 210-17.

Wagstaff, A., Paci, P. and van Doorslaer, E. (1991) 'On the measurement of inequalities in health', *Social Science & Medicine*, vol 33, pp 545-57.

Further reading

Harper, S. and Lynch, J. (2006) *Methods for measuring cancer disparities: A review using data relevant to healthy people 2010 cancer-related objectives*, Washington, DC: National Cancer Institute.

Kunst, A. and Mackenbach, J. (1995) *Measuring socioeconomic inequalities in health*, Copenhagen: World Health Organization, Regional Office for Europe.

Mackenbach, J.P. and Kunst, A.E. (1997) 'Measuring the magnitude of socio-economic inequalities in health: an overview of available measures illustrated with two examples from Europe', *Social Science & Medicine*, vol 44, pp 757-71.

See also: 3.1 Absolute differences; 3.5 Index of Disparity; 3.9 Relative differences

3.3 Gini coefficient

The Gini coefficient is an example of a disproportionality measure of inequality (see **3.6 Measures of average disproportionality**). The Gini coefficient summarises social group differences in health for the entire population, and can be thought of as a measure of association between each social group's share of population, ranked by their health (on the x-axis), and their share of health (on the y-axis). In this sense the Gini coefficient is a 'univariate' measure of inequality and only shows how unevenly health or some other quantity (such as income) is distributed according to population share. It is the most commonly used measure of income inequality (usually in the form where when $\alpha = 2$ and $\beta = 1$, as shown in the formula below) and in this form can also be expressed as the so-called 'Robin Hood Index', which is merely the inverse of the Gini coefficient.

The Gini coefficient takes a value between 0 and 1 (sometimes expressed as a percentage). Zero would indicate perfect equality; the quantity (health, income) is shared equally across the population, so in the income example, every member of the population would have the same income. A value of 1 indicates perfect inequality; in the same example, this would indicate that one individual has all of the income and everyone else has zero income.

Technical detail

The Gini coefficient belongs to a class of inter-individual inequality measures (IID) that summarise all inter-individual differences in health and take the general form:

$$IID(\alpha, \beta) = \frac{\displaystyle\sum_{i=1}^{n} \sum_{j=1}^{n} \left| y_i - y_j \right|^{\alpha}}{2n^2 \mu^{\beta}}$$

where y_i is individual i's health, y_j is individual j's health, μ is the mean health of the population, and n is the number of individuals in the population. When $\alpha = 2$ and $\beta = 1$ the IID is equal to the Gini coefficient. Other weightings of α and β are of course possible. If α is a larger number than 2, it implies giving more weight to bigger inter-individual differences.

Strengths

The measure has been widely used in economics and is well understood as a measure of income inequality.

Limitations

The Gini coefficient is by definition a purely inter-individual inequality indicator and so reflects 'total inequality' in the population. Health inequality researchers are often more interested in between-group inequality and so the interpretation of a Gini coefficient for health is not always clear. Perhaps this is why the Gini coefficient has not been widely used as an indicator of degree of health inequality, although it has been widely used as a measure of income inequality in health studies.

Example

Graphically, the Gini coefficient is the ratio of the area between the line of equality and the Lorenz curve (see the figure below) to the total area of the triangle beneath the line of equality. Because the Gini coefficient is a function of the disproportionality between shares of population and shares of health, one can see that health inequality increases as the Lorenz curve moves further away from the line of equality (that is, as the disproportionality between shares of population and shares of health increases). The Lorenz curve is a graphical representation of the cumulative distribution function of a probability distribution.

Graphical representation of the Gini coefficient of inequality

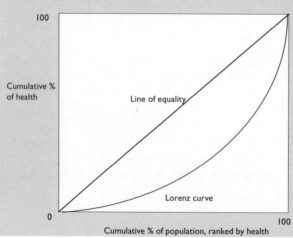

Gakidou and King (2002) have used this inequality measure (with $\alpha = 3$ and $\beta = 1$) to compare total inequality in child survival among 50 countries. A weighting of $\alpha = 3$ implies that the measure should be more sensitive to larger than smaller pairwise deviations between individuals and thus reflects additional concern about larger health differences between individuals.

References

Gakidou, E. and King, G. (2002) 'Measuring total health inequality: adding individual variation to group-level differences', *International Journal for Equity in Health*, vol 1, no 3 (www.equityhealthj.com/content/pdf/1475-9276-1-3.pdf).

Further reading

Harper, S. and Lynch, J. (2006) *Methods for measuring cancer disparities: A review using data relevant to healthy people 2010 cancer-related objectives*, Washington, DC: National Cancer Institute.

Murray, C., Gakidou, E. and Frenk, J. (1999) 'Health inequalities and social group differences: what should we measure?', *Bulletin of the World Health Organization*, no 77, pp 537-43.

Sen, A. and Foster, J. (1997) *On economic inequality*, Oxford: Clarendon Press.

Shkolnikov, V., Andreev, E. and Begun, A. (2003) 'Gini coefficient as a life table function: computation from discrete data, decomposition of differences and empirical examples', *Demographic Research*, vol 8, pp 305-57 (www.demographic-research.org/Volumes/Vol8/11/8-11.pdf).

See also: 3.6 Measures of average disproportionality

3.4 Households Below Average Income (HBAI)

The Households Below Average Income (HBAI) series are official statistics produced by National Statistics and released through the Department for Work and Pensions in an annual report of the same name. The HBAI is a measure that "uses household disposable incomes, adjusted for household size and composition, as a proxy for material living standards or, more precisely, for the level of consumption of goods and services that people could attain given the disposable income of the household in which they live" (HBAI 1994/95–2003/04, p 1). This adjustment for household size and composition, which allows for the comparison of different types of households, is known as 'equivalisation'. It helps to account for the fact that, for example, a household with one working adult and no children is in a different financial situation to a household with the same total income but consisting of two working adults and three dependent children.

The HBAI tells us about the income distribution of the British population by identifying the proportion of households whose income is below various low-income thresholds (for example, below 50% of mean income, or below 60% of median income). This is presented for the whole population, households with children, working-age adults and pensioners. The HBAI report tells us not only about low incomes but also provides information about the entire range of the income distribution. The report also includes Gini coefficients, a measure that can be used to track inequality across the whole income distribution.

The main source of data used for constructing HBAI is the Family Resources Survey, a continuous cross-sectional survey of some 27,000 households in Great Britain, including a boosted sample in Scotland and 2,000 households in Northern Ireland. This is supplemented by data from the British Household Panel Survey, which provides information that tracks individuals and households over time.

Strengths

The main strength of the HBAI series is the range of measures that it includes: for example, it contains information on exit and entry rates into and out of low income; incomes before and after housing costs; lone parents and family size; incomes by regional geography; some data on minority ethnic groups;

and it includes information on the self-employed. The fact that the data are reported annually (there have been 16 reports to date) is also a major strength (although see the comment below). Another strength is that a lot of detail on methodology is provided and data based on small numbers about which there may be some statistical uncertainty are highlighted. Another strong point is that consultation with users is undertaken as to the use and future of the statistics produced.

Limitations

As the HBAI data are based on survey data they will therefore inevitably suffer from sampling error (see the Appendices in each report for detail); non-response, another feature of survey data, is handled through weighting using population totals. The series only covers private households, hence it excludes people in residential institutions (such as nursing homes or university halls) and homeless people. It also under-reports the number of people with very high incomes as well as the magnitude of their income (this is known through comparisons with tax record data). Hence the data will not reflect the full spectrum of incomes in British society.

Although the data are equivalised, the method assumes that all individuals within a household benefit equally from the combined income of the household. Sociological research focusing on gender and marriage relations has shown, for example, that there are many ways of distributing money within the household, and many variations can be found even within one type of household, such as cohabiting couples (Vogler, 2005).

Another potential weakness is that there are changes in the methodology that have implications for making valid comparisons over time, for example, in the 2003/04 figures the grossing regime methodology was changed (due to changes in population estimates since the 2001 Census). In this case a revised historic series was also produced, but in general it is worth being very careful about reading the technical notes to make sure that you are making valid comparisons over time.

Discussion point

Selected key findings from the HBAI statistics, 2003/04

- Benefits together with tax credits were the main source of income for the bottom quintile in 2003/04 whereas earnings were the main source for the other four quintiles.
- In 2003/04, individuals in workless families were much more likely to live in low-income households than those with one or more adults in full-time work.
- Families with children, particularly lone-parent families, were more at risk of low income in 2003/04 than their childless counterparts.
- Women had a slightly higher risk of low income than men in 2003/04.
- In 2003/04, individuals living in households headed by a member of a minority ethnic community were more likely to live in low-income households. This was particularly the case for households headed by someone of Pakistani/Bangladeshi ethnic origin.
- Individuals in families containing one or more disabled people were more likely to live in low-income households in 2003/04 than those in families with no disabled person.

Source: HBAI (1994/95–2003/04, p 6)

References

HBAI reports are available at the Department for Work and Pensions website:
www.dwp.gov.uk/asd/hbai/hbai2005/contents.asp

Vogler, C. (2005) 'Cohabiting couples: rethinking money in the household at the beginning of the twenty first century', *The Sociological Review*, vol 53, no 1, pp 1-29.

Weblinks

Family Resources Survey:
www.dwp.gov.uk/asd/frs

British Household Panel Survey:
http://iserwww.essex.ac.uk/ulsc/bhps/

See also: 1.8 Living standards; 2.16 Income; 3.3 Gini coefficient

3.5 Index of Disparity

The Index of Disparity is the average deviation of group rates from a chosen reference rate. It summarises the difference between several group rates and a reference rate and expresses the summed differences as a proportion of the reference rate.

Technical detail

This measure was formally introduced by Pearcy and Keppel (2002) and is calculated as:

$$\left(\sum_{j=1}^{J-1} \left| r_j - r_{ref} \right| / J \right) / r_{ref} \times 100$$

where r_j indicates the measure of health status in the jth group, r_{ref} is the health status indicator in the reference group population, and J is the number of groups compared. While in principle any reference group may be chosen, Pearcy and Keppel (2002) recommend the best group rate as the comparison since that represents the rate desirable for all groups to achieve.

Strengths

The Index of Disparity is simple to calculate summary measure that represents the literal definition of 'inequality as difference' among groups. It can be used for any sort of social groupings, such as occupational social class, without the need for any ranking.

Limitations

This measure does not consider the population size of any group. If each group is given the same weight contributed by any other group, then population groups comprising greater numbers of individuals are effectively down-weighted. Thus, if social group A contained 10,000 individuals and social group B contained 100,000 individuals, the individuals in group B would be contributing 1/10th of the information on health inequality contributed by those individuals in group A. Calculating a weighted version of the Index of Disparity is a simple adaptation of the formula. However, the decision to weight or not relies on making value judgements about the relative importance of considering groups as entities versus individuals in calculating this indicator of inequality. This is a rather more complicated task. The reasons for a decision to use a weighted or unweighted index should, however, be made explicit.

Example

Using total rate across all groups as the reference rate

Calculating the Index of Disparity

Social group	Rate	| Group-total|
A	6.0	1.2
B	13.9	6.7
C	5.8	1.4
D	5.5	1.7
E	9.3	2.1
Total rate	7.2	–
Σ | Group-total |		13.1
Σ | Group-total |/5 groups		2.62
Mean deviation/reference point = (Σ | Group-total |/5)/total		0.36

The average inequality across the five groups is 0.36 or 36% of the total population rate.

References

Pearcy, J. and Keppel, K. (2002) 'A summary measure of health disparity', *Public Health Reports*, vol 117, pp 273-80.

Further reading

Keppel, K., Pearcy, J. and Wagener, D. (2002) *Trends in racial and ethnic-specific rates for the health status indicators: United States, 1990-98*, Healthy People 2000 Statistical Notes, no 23, 2002-1237, Hyattsville, MD: National Center for Health Statistics.

Keppel, K., Pamuk, E., Lynch, J., Carter-Pokras, O., Kim, I., Mays, V., Pearcy, J., Schoenbach, V. and Weissman, J. (2005) 'Methodological issues in measuring health disparities. National Center for Health Statistics', *Vital Health Statistics*, Series 2,141, pp 1-16.

See also: 3.2 Dissimilarity Index

3.6 Measures of average disproportionality

When describing health inequalities, public health researchers and policy makers often use what might be called the 'language of disproportionality'. For example, in the context of arguing for the importance of measuring health inequalities between socially meaningful population groups, Braveman and colleagues (2000) discussed how a 'disproportionate share' of ill health was carried by the socially disadvantaged. Terms such as 'disproportionate share' and 'unequal burden' are important qualifiers because they communicate the ethical notions inherent in the collective concerns over health inequalities. That is, they capture the notion that it is unfair that some groups experience more ill health than others; a just distribution of health implies that ill health should be experienced proportionately by different social groups. Measures of average disproportionality are therefore a group of metrics that can be used to assess the extent of this 'disproportionality'.

Technical detail

For each social group j we can define a health ratio as the ratio of a measure of health y in the jth group, to that of the mean of y for the whole population, so that $r_j = Y_j / \overline{Y}$ for each group. Note that this makes such measures relative rather than absolute inequality indicators. In this framework, measures of inequality take the general form

$$I = \sum_j p_j f(r_j)$$

where p_j is group j's proportion of the total population and $f(r_j)$ is some disproportionality function of the ratio $r_j = Y_j / \overline{Y}$. It should be clear that these measures are population weighted, since each group's disproportionality function $f(r_j)$ is multiplied by their population share p_j. Measures of this family of inequality indicators differ only because they implement different disproportionality functions $(f(r_j))$.

Strengths

One of the appealing features of disproportionality measures is that they provide a direct correspondence between the commonly used language of health inequality in terms of 'unequal burden' with the direct operationalisation of the measurement. These measures account for population size and can be used with ranked and non-ranked data. Some can be depicted graphically, which aids interpretation (see also **3.8 Relative Concentration Index (RCI)**).

Limitations

These are sophisticated measures that have not been very widely used and are somewhat complicated to calculate. As such they are relatively unfamiliar to both researchers and policy makers, which may in the short term make them more difficult to communicate.

Example

The figure shows a graphical depiction of the concept of 'disproportionality' using data on all deaths in the US, by gender and education, for the year 2000. Among males, those with less than 12 years of education bear a disproportionate burden of all deaths, as they account for 24% of all male deaths but account for only 13% of the male population. Conversely, males with more than 12 years of education account for 55% of the total population, but only 32% of all deaths. Disproportionality measures of inequality summarise these differences (in various ways) between shares of population and shares of health.

Graphical example of the 'disproportionality' of deaths and population, by gender and education

'Disproportionality'

Shares of all deaths and population, by gender and education, 2000

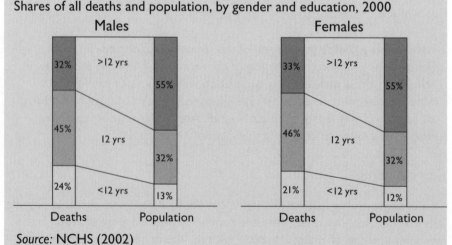

Source: NCHS (2002)

Many commonly used measures of inequality may be conveniently expressed as measures of average disproportionality. The table shows some commonly used statistical measures and their disproportionality functions. The table makes clear that the measures differ only in how they express the ratio of shares of health and shares of population.

Commonly used disproportionality functions

Index name	Disproportionality function
Squared coefficient of variation (CV^2)	$(r_j - 1)^2$
Gini index (G)	Individual-level data: $\lvert r_i - r_j \rvert / 2$
	Grouped data: $r_j(q_j - Q_j)$, where q_j is the proportion of the total population in groups less healthy than group j, and Q_j is the proportion of the total population in groups healthier than group j (ie, $p_j + q_j + Q_j = 1$)
Relative Concentration Index (RCI)	Same as for G, but groups are ranked by social group position instead of by health, so that q_j is the proportion of the total population in groups less advantaged than group j, and Q_j is the proportion of the total population in groups more advantaged than group j (ie, $p_j + q_j + Q_j = 1$)
Theil Index (T)	$r_j \ln(r_j)$
Mean logarithmic deviation (MLD)	$\ln(1 / r_j) = -\ln(r_j)$
Variance of log-health (VarLog)	$[\ln r_j - \Sigma(\ln r_j)]^2$

Note: Adapted from Firebaugh (2003)

References

Braveman, P., Krieger, N. and Lynch, J. (2000) 'Health inequalities and social inequalities in health', *Bulletin of the World Health Organization*, vol 78, pp 232-4.

Firebaugh, G. (2003) *The new geography of global income inequality*, Cambridge, MA: Harvard University Press.

NCHS (National Center for Health Statistics) (2002) 'Deaths: final data for 2000', *National Vital Statistics Reports*, vol 50, no 15.

Further reading

Harper, S. and Lynch, J. (2006) *Methods for measuring cancer disparities: A review using data relevant to healthy people 2010 cancer-related objectives*, Washington, DC: National Cancer Institute.

See also: 3.3 Gini coefficient; 3.8 Relative Concentration Index (RCI); 3.13 Theil Index and mean log deviation

3.7 Range

The range of inequality is one of the commonest measures of inequality used in the health inequality literature, and compares the experience of the top and bottom socioeconomic groups. When comparing areas, the range can be used to compare the area with the worst outcome (such as the highest level of deprivation) with the area with the best outcome (the lowest level of deprivation). These comparisons can be made with either absolute (risk difference) or relative differences (ratios).

Strengths

The range provides a measure of the complete extent of inequality by comparing the most extreme groups. This can be an eye-catching and effective means of communicating the extent of inequalities.

Limitations

No account is taken of what is happening in the groups or areas that are not at the extremes. It is possible that the gap between the top and bottom may be extreme while there is little difference between the intermediate groups. Likewise, when looking at changes in inequality over time, only looking at the range may suggest that inequalities at the extremes are increasing while in the intermediate groups they are stable or even decreasing. No account is taken of the proportion of the population in the extreme groups. This is particularly problematic if the extreme groups represent only a small proportion of the total population, in which case the outcomes for the majority of the population do not contribute to the measure of inequality, and the estimate of inequality will be imprecise and influenced by random variation.

Example

The UK 'Black Report' on socioeconomic inequalities in health reported that men and women in social class V (manual workers) had a 2.5 times greater chance of dying before reaching retirement age than men and women in social class I (professionals).

Source: Townsend (1982)

References
Townsend, P. (1982) *Inequalities in health: The Black Report*, Harmondsworth: Penguin.

See also: 3.1 Absolute differences; 3.6 Measures of average disproportionality; 3.9 Relative differences

3.8 Relative Concentration Index (RCI)

The Relative Concentration Index (RCI), an example of a disproportionality measure of inequality (see **3.6 Measures of average disproportionality**), measures the extent to which health or illness is concentrated among particular social groups. The RCI is calculated in a similar way to the Gini coefficient, but it results from a 'bivariate' rather than 'univariate' distribution of health and social group ranking. In the same way that the Gini coefficient is derived from the Lorenz curve, the RCI is similarly derived from a health concentration curve, where the population is first ordered by social group status (rather than by health status as for the Gini) and the cumulative percentage of the population according to social group rank (on the x-axis) is then plotted against their share of total health (on the y-axis). The RCI may only be used with social groups that have an inherent ranking, such as income or education groups.

Technical detail

The general formula for the RCI for grouped data is given by Kakwani and colleagues (1997) as:

$$RCI = \frac{2}{\mu}\left[\sum\nolimits_{j=1}^{J} p_j \mu_j R_j\right] - 1$$

where p_j is the group's population share, μ_j is the group's mean health, and R_j is the relative rank of the jth socioeconomic group, which is defined as:

$$R_j = \sum\nolimits_{j=1}^{J} p_\gamma - \frac{1}{2}p_j$$

where p_y is the cumulative share of the population up to and including group j and p_j is the share of the population in group j. R_j essentially indicates the cumulative share of the population up to the midpoint of each group interval, similar to the categorisation used for the Slope Index of Inequality (SII) (see **3.11**). In fact, the RCI has a specific mathematical relationship with the SII, such that,

$$HCI = 2\operatorname{var}(x)(\beta / \mu)$$

where β is the slope parameter identified in the equation for the SII.

Wagstaff (2002) has also derived a method for incorporating a society's degree of aversion to inequality into the RCI, which he calls the 'Extended' Concentration Index (2002). The aversion parameter changes the weight attached to the health of different socioeconomic groups. The formula for this extended version of the RCI for grouped data is:

$$HCI(v) = 1 - \frac{v}{\mu} \sum_{j=1}^{J} p_j \mu_j (1 - R_j)^{v-1}$$

where v is the 'aversion parameter' and the other quantities are defined as above. Setting $v = 1$ weights every group's health equally, and setting $v = 2$ gives the standard RCI defined above. Generally, the weight attached to the health of lower socioeconomic groups increases and the weight attached to the health of higher socioeconomic groups decreases as v increases.

The Absolute Concentration Index (ACI) measures the extent to which health or illness is concentrated among particular social groups on the absolute scale. The absolute version of the concentration index is calculated by multiplying the RCI by the mean (μ) of the health variable:

$$ACI = \mu RCI$$

Strengths

One of the reasons the RCI and ACI (and, by extension, the SII and the Relative Index of Inequality [RII]) are favoured by some is that they specifically reflect the socioeconomic aspects of inequalities in health. That is, a health gradient where health worsens among groups of lower social rank results in a positive RCI, whereas an upward health gradient results in a negative RCI. The RCI can be graphed to aid quick interpretation (see the figure below) and it reflects the population size of different social groups, unlike range measures of inequality such as the rate or prevalence ratios.

Limitations

The RCI requires social groups to be hierarchically ordered and so cannot be used with social groups categorised by gender or race/ethnicity. It has not been widely used in health inequalities research and so may be more unfamiliar and initially more difficult to interpret. As the RCI becomes more widely used these limitations will lessen.

Graphical representation of the health concentration curve

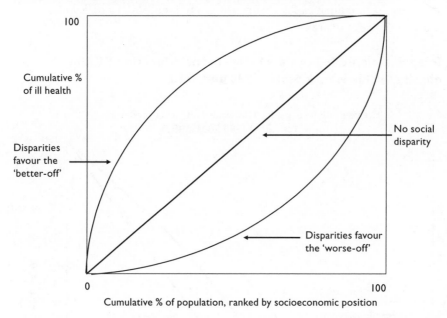

Example

The figure above gives a graphical representation of the RCI curve. Note the similarity with the Lorenz curve that illustrates the Gini coefficient (see **3.3**). The two curves, and thus the Gini coefficient and the RCI, are calculated similarly, the only difference being the ordering of the social groups. In the case of the Gini coefficient, the social groups are ordered by their health status (lowest to highest), regardless of their social group ranking, while for the RCI the social groups are ordered by their ranking in terms of their social group, such as years of education, regardless of their health status. It is important to note that, because the RCI incorporates information on both health and social group status, the concentration curve may lie either above or below the line of equality. Since the y-axis in the figure is now the share of 'ill health' rather than health, the curve lies above the line of equality.

The graphical depiction of change in the RCI below clearly shows that educational inequality in obesity between 1990 and 2002 decreased since the health concentration curve in 2002 is closer to the line of equality than in 1990. This ability to plot the curves may make this measure attractive for communicating changes in health inequality to policy makers and stakeholders (Harper and Lynch, 2006).

Graphical depiction of the change in the education RCI for obesity for New York State, 1990 and 2002

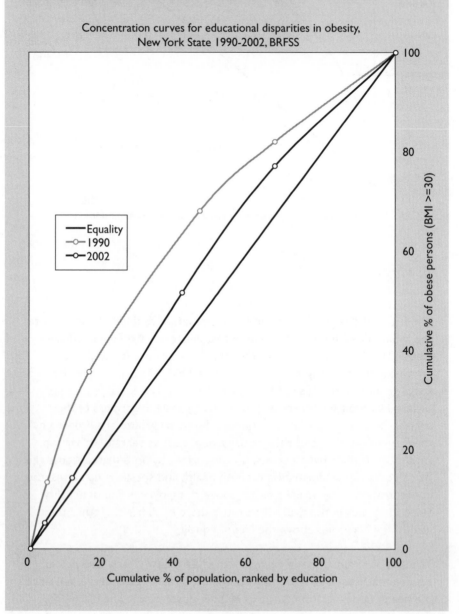

Concentration curves for educational disparities in obesity,
New York State 1990-2002, BRFSS

References

Harper, S. and Lynch J. (2007) 'Trends in socioeconomic inequalities in adult health behaviors among US states, 1990-2004', *Public Health Reports*, vol 122, no 2, pp 177-89.

Wagstaff, A. (2002) 'Inequality aversion, health inequalities and health achievement', *Journal of Health Economics*, vol 21, pp 627-41.

Further reading

Kakwani, N., Wagstaff, A. and Vandoorslaer, E. (1997) 'Socioeconomic inequalities in health: measurement, computation, and statistical inference', *Journal of Econometrics*, vol 77, pp 87-103.

Wagstaff, A. (2000) 'Socioeconomic inequalities in child mortality: comparisons across nine developing countries, *Bulletin of the World Health Organization*, vol 78, pp 19-29.

Wagstaff, A. (2002) 'Inequality aversion, health inequalities and health achievement', *Journal of Health Economics*, vol 21, pp 627-41.

Wagstaff, A. (2003) 'Child health on a dollar a day: some tentative cross-country comparisons', *Social Science & Medicine*, vol 57, pp 1529-38.

See also: 3.3 Gini coefficient; 3.6 Measures of average disproportionality; 3.10 Relative Index of Inequality (RII); 3.11 Slope Index of Inequality (SII)

3.9   Relative differences

Both relative and absolute differences are measures of the strength of association between social group differences in health since they examine the absolute or relative difference in an outcome (for example, health or disease status) by categories of an exposure (for example, social class groups). A relative difference (also known as relative effect or relative risk) refers to the outcome of an exposure, expressed as the ratio between means, odds, rates, risk, and so on, as opposed to being expressed as a difference between these (see **3.1 Absolute differences**). The exposure of interest might be a measure of socioeconomic position (SEP), sex, ethnicity, age, geographical area or time period. Unlike absolute differences a relative difference does not depend on the prevalence of the outcome and is usually more stable between populations.

Strengths

The relative risk is usually a better indicator of disease aetiology (than measures of absolute difference), and is therefore often used in epidemiology.

Limitations

Relative differences dominate health inequalities research, but there is no rule that inequality should only be assessed in relative terms. Indeed, there is much debate about whether inequalities should be expressed as absolute or relative differences (Wagstaff et al, 1991; Mackenbach and Kunst, 1997; Ebrahim, 2002; Oliver et al, 2002; Low and Low, 2005; Shaw et al, 2005), and arguments for one or another may be driven to some extent by the results produced and by the particular message the researchers want to communicate. Relative and absolute differences represent different aspects of the data and both are valid measurements. In epidemiology, relative risks are taken as better indices of aetiological effect, absolute differences as better indices of public health importance. Inequalities in health have relevance to both aetiology and public health and ideally both absolute and relative differences (or results that would allow both to be calculated) should be presented in research and reports of inequality.

Example

In the UK the *Independent Inquiry into Inequalities in Health* (referred to as the Acheson Inquiry) all-cause mortality was presented by different social classes so that absolute and relative differences could be calculated. All-cause mortality in UK men aged 20-64 years in 1991-93 was 806 per 100,000 for those in social class V and 280 per 100,000 for those in social class I. The relative difference in mortality is 2.88 (806/280) (which compares to an absolute difference of 526 per 100,000).

Note: Social class here refers to the UK Registrar General's classification of occupational Social Classes. Note also that the comparison between the two extreme groups of social class is sometimes referred to as the range of inequality.

Source: Acheson (1998)

References

Acheson, Sir Donald (1998) *Independent Inquiry into Inequalities in Health*, London: The Stationery Office.

Ebrahim, S. (2002) 'Addressing health inequalities', *Lancet,* vol 360, p 1691.

Low, A. and Low, A. (2005) 'Health inequalities under New Labour: relative rather than absolute gaps are more important over time and place', *BMJ*, vol 330, p 1507.

Mackenbach, J.P. and Kunst, A.E (1997) 'Measuring the magnitude of socio-economic inequalities in health: an overview of available measures illustrated with two examples from Europe', *Social Science & Medicine*, vol 44, pp 757-71.

Oliver, A., Healey, A. and Le Grand, J. (2002) 'Addressing health inequalities', *Lancet*, vol 360, pp 565-7.

Shaw, M., Davey Smith, G. and Dorling, D. (2005) 'Health inequalities under New Labour: authors' reply', *BMJ*, vol 330, pp 1507-8.

Wagstaff, A., Paci, P. and van Doorslaer, E. (1991) 'On the measurement of inequalities in health', *Social Science & Medicine*, vol 33, pp 545-57.

Further reading

Regidor, E. (2004) 'Measures of health inequalities: part 2', *Journal of Epidemiology and Community Health*, vol 58, pp 900-3.

See also: 2.26 Occupational social class – Registrar General's social classes (RGSC); 3.1 Absolute differences; 3.7 Range; 4.14 Populations

3.10 Relative Index of Inequality (RII)

Once a measure of socioeconomic position (SEP) has been obtained, for categorical measures (with at least three categories) the association between the SEP measure and the outcome of interest can be assessed using the Relative Index of Inequality (RII). The RII is useful when making comparisons of the magnitude of the association between the same SEP measure and outcomes in different populations (such as different birth cohorts or populations from different geographical locations), or when making comparisons in the magnitude of effect of different measures of SEP with the same outcome of interest. This is because it takes account of differences in the proportions of participants in each category for the different populations or different measurements. Examples of its use include comparing the effect of childhood and adult social class on heart disease, or the effect of educational attainment and occupational social class on smoking behaviour (Wagstaff et al, 1991; Kunst and Mackenbach, 1994; Mackenbach and Kunst, 1997).

Technical detail

The measure of SEP is first converted to a score between 0 (the lowest SEP) and 1 (the highest). The score is weighted according to the population in each SEP group by calculating the midpoint of the proportion of the population in each category. For example, again using the UK Registrar General's Occupational Social Classes, if 10% of the study participants were in the lowest occupational social class (V) and 15% were in the next lowest category (IV):

- participants in social class V would be assigned a score of 0.05 (0.10/2). This score reflects that 95% of the population have a higher SEP than the average person in this group;
- those in social class IV would be allocated a score of 0.175 (0.10 + (0.15/2)), and so on for each social class.

The RII is then obtained by regressing each of these SEP scores on the outcome, using the appropriate generalised regression model (linear, logistic, Poisson) for the data. The regression coefficient from this model is the Slope Index of Inequality (SII) (see **3.11**). The RII is the SII divided by the mean value of the outcome measure:

$$RII = SII / \mu$$

Strengths

The virtue of the RII is that it is directly interpretable in terms of outcome difference between the lowest value (score 0, the hypothetically worst-off person in the population) and highest value (score 1, the hypothetically best-off person in the population) of whichever SEP indicator is used. In some respects it is comparable to the familiar (in epidemiology, health service research, psychology and statistics) practice of standardising any continuous exposures (risk factors) in the form of standard deviation units. Since all of the measurements of RII are on the same scale it simplifies comparisons between the effects of different measures of SEP (or the same measure in different populations). Estimates based on the RII are also less influenced by extremes of the exposure distribution.

Limitations

Although the RII puts different measures of SEP onto the same scale this is a mathematical process and does not mean that different measures (such as occupational social class and educational achievement) within the same population or the same measure in different populations have the same meaning. When using the RII to make such comparisons one has to interpret results based on a sensible discussion of how the meaning of different measures is likely to have affected the results. While continuous measures of SEP can be categorised to generate an RII, it is not useful to estimate an RII for a binary measure of SEP (such as owning/not owning a car), since irrespective of the proportions in the two groups the difference between them will always be the same. This measure is also based on the assumption that everyone in the lowest SEP group is worse off than everyone in all the groups above, which is unrealistic.

The RII and the **Slope Index of Inequality (SII)** (see **3.11**) depend on having a social group classification scheme that is hierarchical. This seems uncontroversial with respect to education and income, but social group classifications based on occupation may be somewhat more challenging, because there is inherently more ambiguity in the ranking of occupations. The RII and SII cannot be used for assessing health inequality among social groups such as ethnic or gender groups, which have no inherent ordering.

Example

The figure shows the predicted slope for income-related inequality (based on income-to-poverty ratio) in smoking. The absolute difference in smoking prevalence from the top (score=1) to the bottom (score=0) of the income hierarchy is 18.1% (this is the SII). The RII is the SII divided by the mean of the outcome measure (in this case, the average smoking rate of 24.6%).

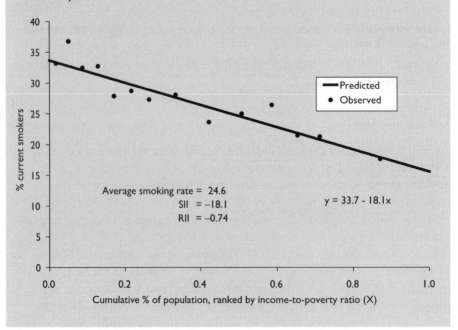

Average smoking rate = 24.6
SII = −18.1
RII = −0.74

y = 33.7 - 18.1x

References

Kunst, A.E. and Mackenbach, J.P. (1994) 'The size of mortality differences associated with educational level in nine industrialized countries', *American Journal of Public Health*, vol 84, pp 932-7.

Mackenbach, J.P. and Kunst, A.E. (1997) 'Measuring the magnitude of socio-economic inequalities in health: an overview of available measures illustrated with two examples from Europe', *Social Science & Medicine*, vol 44, no 6, pp 757-71.

Wagstaff, A., Paci, P. and van Doorslaer, E. (1991) 'On the measurement of inequalities in health', *Social Science & Medicine*, vol 33, pp 545-57.

See also: 2.26 Occupational social class – Registrar General's social classes (RGSC); 3.1 Absolute differences; 3.9 Relative differences; 3.11 Slope Index of Inequality (SII)

3.11 Slope Index of Inequality (SII)

The Slope Index of Inequality (SII), which was introduced by Preston et al (1981), is a measure of absolute inequality. It is derived via regression of mean health within a particular social group on the mean relative rank of social groups (see Technical detail). To calculate relative rank, the social groups are first ordered from lowest to highest. The population of each social group category covers a range in the cumulative distribution of the population, and so is given a score based on the midpoint of their range in the cumulative distribution in the population according to the group rank (see Example). The SII therefore represents the hypothetical absolute difference in outcome (for example, mortality rate) between the bottom and the top of the measure of socioeconomic position (SEP) on the basis of the regression model and is similar to the Relative Index of Inequality (RII), but reports absolute instead of relative differences between the hypothetically worst-off and hypothetically best-off person in the population.

Example

		Ranking social groups as cumulative proportions of the population		
Social group	%	Cumulative %	Range	Midpoint
1	5.66	5.66	0.0–5.66	2.83
2	10.65	16.31	5.67–16.31	10.99
3	34.10	50.42	16.32–50.42	33.37
4	25.95	76.37	50.43–76.37	63.40
5	23.63	100.0	76.38–100.0	88.19

Thus, social group 1 comprises 5.66% of the population and occupies from 0–5.66% of the cumulative proportion of the population. It is assigned the midpoint in the cumulative distribution of 2.83. Social group 2 occupies the next 10.65% in the cumulative distribution and it is assigned the midpoint of its place in the cumulative distribution of 10.99, and so on. This allows all social groups to be assigned their relative rank in the population and these values are then regressed against the mean level of health in each social group.

Technical detail

The regression equation is specified as follows:

$$\bar{y}_j = \beta_0 + \beta_1 \bar{R}_j$$

where j indexes social group, $\bar{y}_j$ is the average health status and $\bar{R}_j$ the average relative ranking of social group j in the cumulative distribution of the population, β_0 is the estimated health status of a hypothetical person at the bottom of the social group hierarchy (that is, a person whose relative rank R_j in the social group distribution is 0), and β_1 is the difference in average health status between the hypothetical person at the bottom of the social group distribution and the hypothetical person at the top (that is, $R_j=0$ vs $R_j=1$). Because the relative rank variable is based on the cumulative proportions of the population (from 0 to 1), a 'one-unit' change in relative rank is equivalent to moving from the bottom to the top of the social group distribution. Because this regression is run on grouped data (as opposed to individual data) it is estimated via *weighted* least squares, with the weights equal to the population share p_j of group j. The coefficient β_1 is the SII, and is interpreted as the absolute difference in health status between the bottom and top of the social group distribution.

References

Preston, S., Haines, M. and Pamuk E. (1981) 'Effects of industrialization and urbanization on mortality in developed countries', in International Union for the Scientific Study of Population (ed) *International Population Conference, Manila, 1981: Solicited Papers*, Leige: Ordina Editions, pp 233-54.

Further reading

Davey Smith, G., Dorling, D., Mitchell, R. and Shaw, M. (2002) 'Health inequalities in Britain: continuing increases up to the end of the 20th century', *Journal of Epidemiology and Community Health*, vol 56, pp 434-5.

Harper, S. and Lynch, J. (2006) *Methods for measuring cancer disparities: A review using data relevant to healthy people 2010 cancer-related objectives*, Washington, DC: National Cancer Institute.

Kunst, A. and Mackenbach, J. (1994) 'International variation in the size of mortality differences associated with occupational status', *International Journal of Epidemiology*, vol 23, pp 742-50.

Pamuk, E. (1988) 'Social-class inequality in infant mortality in England and Wales from 1921 to 1980', *European Journal of Population*, vol 4, pp 1-21.

See also: 3.10 Relative Index of Inequality (RII)

3.12 Standardised outcomes

Standardisation is a procedure for adjusting outcomes (such as prevalence and incidence rates) to take account of differences in the composition of populations, in terms of population characteristics such as age structure and gender mix. For example, one would expect crude rates (rates that have been calculated without taking the population structure into account) of coronary heart disease to be greater in a population with a larger proportion of elderly individuals than one with a predominance of young individuals. Once a measure has been age-sex standardised it means that differences in rates between populations cannot be explained by differences in their age or sex structure, and must therefore be explained by other factors. Most analyses of routine data sources that present rates age-standardise them.

There area two approaches commonly used for standardisation:

- direct standardisation
- indirect standardisation, usually expressed as a standardised ratio.

Both methods are based on calculated weighted averages for rates specifically for age, sex and sometimes other potential confounding variables (although it is more common to use other procedures, such as multivariable analysis, covered in standard epidemiology textbooks, for adjusting for other potential confounding factors).

Direct standardisation

The direct method averages specific rates in a study population using as weights the population distribution of a specified population. This 'reference' or 'standard' population could be a theoretical standard, for example, the World Health Organization (WHO) European standard population (see www.who.int). Alternatively, if assessing rates in a subsample of a population in which distributions for the whole population are known, these may be used. For example, the population of England may be used as the reference population to directly standardise rates for the population of a local authority. The standardised rate here represents what the crude rate would have been in the study population if the population had the same distribution as the standard population with respect to the variables for which the adjustment or standardisation was carried out. For example, if a local authority's all-cause mortality rate is age-sex standardised using the English population as the reference population, the directly standardised rate represents the mortality rate the local authority would have *if it had the same age-sex structure as the English population.*

Technical detail

Directly age-sex standardised rate = $(\sum p_k m_k) / \sum p_k$

Where:

- k = sex/age group (for example <1, 1-4, 5-9, 10-14, 15-19 ... 85+ for females and males);
- p_k is the population in sex/age group k in the reference population;
- m_k is the observed mortality rate (for example, deaths per million persons) in sex/age group k in the study population.

Directly standardised rates can be easily calculated in spreadsheets or statistical computer packages.

Example

Worked example of calculation of directly standardised mortality rates from circulatory diseases for men aged 35-74 years for England and Wales (1921-41). Rates standardised to the 1991 WHO European standard population

Year	Age-specific mortality rates								Directly age standardised rate 35-74
	35-39	40-44	45-49	50-54	55-59	60-64	65-69	70-74	
1921	75.1	107.1	162.1	299.8	522.4	888.7	1,567.0	2,568.0	566.5
1922	75.5	112.5	174.5	299.8	534.8	985.9	1,714.3	2,827.8	611.2
1923	67.2	101.8	169.4	278.0	520.1	917.6	1,667.5	2,611.9	576.7
1924	62.3	100.4	167.3	285.2	533.0	968.8	1,714.2	2,840.5	602.7
1925	55.6	98.1	169.9	285.3	548.3	940.6	1,797.5	2,895.2	611.5
1926	59.0	90.1	169.8	281.9	522.8	935.4	1,770.9	2,797.1	597.7
1927	57.8	102.8	174.5	295.4	545.5	1,024.8	1,814.1	3,061.3	635.9
1928	59.5	98.4	177.6	304.2	537.2	1,024.1	1,860.8	3,173.6	647.5
1929	58.2	109.3	189.2	329.0	589.0	1,107.6	2,028.5	3,552.7	709.7
1930	58.3	99.7	174.7	309.7	562.6	1,056.2	1,812.6	3,318.5	660.0
1931	60.7	102.8	182.0	329.9	598.1	1,093.7	2,036.1	3,554.2	708.5
1932	56.1	98.1	183.7	328.3	594.3	1,067.1	2,033.8	3,602.7	706.7
1933	58.2	100.0	190.8	343.5	611.7	1,052.3	1,995.9	3,581.7	706.7
1934	56.9	96.9	187.3	344.2	617.1	1,101.2	2,005.1	3,600.2	713.6
1935	56.3	101.0	190.2	357.3	628.0	1,121.9	2,020.0	3,581.5	720.3
1936	60.5	104.3	198.4	385.5	664.0	1,214.5	2,084.4	3,814.4	762.6
1937	56.6	101.9	194.1	383.2	663.0	1,234.8	2,084.9	3,794.8	761.4
1938	52.8	98.9	188.5	372.9	659.4	1,197.7	2,078.3	3,671.1	744.9
1939	53.3	104.7	203.1	407.8	727.4	1,276.3	2,186.1	3,872.7	793.3
1940	58.4	98.1	194.9	378.8	692.4	1,245.9	2,167.0	3,717.5	767.7
1941	56.5	89.8	177.5	336.5	618.1	1,105.7	1,939.6	3,283.6	684.1

The table above shows an example of the calculation of directly standardised mortality rates (per 100,000) for circulatory diseases among men aged 35-74 years in England and Wales for the years 1921-41. The age-specific mortality rates were calculated using data from the Office for National Statistics (ONS) 20th century mortality CD-ROM and so use death certificate mortality data for the numerator and mid-year population estimates from census, births, deaths and migration data. The age-standardised rates are calculated using the 1991 WHO European standard population (which has a population of 7,000 for each age group 35-39, 40-44, 45-49, 50-54; 6,000 for the age group 55-59; 5,000 for the age group 60-64; 4,000 for the group 65-69 and 3,000 for the age group 70-74). For example, with reference to the equation presented in the Technical detail box, the age-standardised rate for 1921 is calculated as:

$$[(75.10*7,000)+(107.11*7,000)+(162.13*7,000)+(299.79*7,000)+ (522.38*6,000)+(888.69*5,000)+(1567.0*4,000)+(2568.0*3,000)] \div [(7,000+7,000+,000+7,000+6,000+5,000+4,000+3,000)]$$

The standardised rate of 566.5 deaths per 100,000 is the rate that would have been seen in 1921 if the population age structure of males in England and Wales was the same as that of males in the 1991 WHO European standard population. Since all rates in the table are standardised to this same reference population, it is possible to observe the trend in circulatory disease mortality having accounted for any changes in the age structure of England and Wales between 1921 and 1941.

Indirect standardisation

As described previously, direct standardisation produces the death (or disease/illness) rate that would be expected in the study population if it had the *same age/sex structure as the reference population*. In contrast, indirect standardisation produces an estimate of the number of events (usually deaths) that would be expected in the study population if it had the *same age/sex-specific death rates as a reference population*.

The indirect method of standardisation is used to compare study populations for which the age/sex-specific rates in the study populations are either statistically unstable (based on small numbers) or unknown. For this calculation all we need to know is the total number of deaths (all ages) in our study area and its population structure (the number of males and females in each

5- or 10-year age band). Using the known age- and sex-specific mortality rates in a standard reference population, we can then allocate the expected number of deaths in our study population to the appropriate age/sex groups. The ratio of observed events (such as total deaths in the study area) to expected events for the study population is the standardised mortality (or morbidity) ratio, or SMR. In studying time trends, the standard population would typically be one of the years studied, often the first year of the period that the study covers.

Technical detail

$$SMR = 100 * (observed\ deaths/expected\ deaths)$$

Where:

- k = sex/age group (for example 0, 1-4, 5-9, 10-14, 15-19 ... 85+ for males and females)
- expected deaths = $\sum p_k m_k$ where p_k is the population in sex/age group k in the study population; m_k is the mortality rate in sex/age group k for the standard population.

Note that in a time series study, p_k would be the population in sex/age group k in the year of interest ('study population'), and m_k the mortality rate in sex/age group k for the reference year ('reference population').

Example

Example of indirect age standardisation

The table below shows the calculation of a SMR for all-cause mortality in a deprived area of England (this is compared to the standard population of England as a whole).

Calculation of male SMR in a deprived area of England compared to England as a whole

Age group	No of subjects in study population (deprived area of interest)	Death rate (per 1,000 per year) in reference population (England) for people in this age group	Expected number of deaths in study population
0-20	10,000	0.1	1
21-30	4,500	0.5	2.25
31-40	4,000	0.5	2
41-50	3,000	0.7	2.1
51-60	2,000	3.0	6
61+	500	10.0	5
Total	24,000		18.35

Thus in our study population we would expect 18.35 deaths over the one-year period. In fact 50 deaths were observed.

Calculate the indirect SMR = ((observed/expected)*100)

Indirect SMR = (50/18.35)*100 = 272

Commonly SMRs are presented, but these can be used to estimate an indirectly adjusted rate. This is calculated by multiplying the crude mortality rate in the standard population by the SMR (the SMR must be expressed as a proportion here rather than a percentage). In the example, the crude rate in the reference population was 1.5 per 1,000, and the SMR was 272 (2.72 as a proportion), so the indirectly standardised rate for the area of interest would be:

$$(1.5 \text{ per } 1,000) \times 2.72 = 4.08 \text{ per } 1,000$$

Indirect compared to direct standardisation

Indirect	Direct
No need to know age/sex-specific death rates in study population – only its age/sex structure	Need to know age/sex-specific death rates in study population
The choice of reference population influences ratio (but less sensitive than direct method)	Choice of reference population important
Less of a concern if there are small numbers of events within particular age groups	Unstable if age-specific rates are based on small number of events

For both methods it is important to be aware that the simple summary measure obtained may over-simplify quite complex age- and sex-specific variation in mortality patterns in the study population. For example, an SMR of 100 for coronary heart disease (suggesting a similar mortality rate in the study population as in the standard population) may occur in the context of higher than expected coronary heart disease mortality in younger people (and hence greater years of life lost) and a lower than expected mortality in the older age groups. It is best to compare age-specific mortality rates within each age stratum, first with those of the reference population and then test for heterogeneity.

It is also important to recognise that the choice of reference population will affect the actual standardised rate obtained for each study group (defined by geographical area or time), whether direct or indirect standardisation is undertaken. A weighted mean is being calculated with either method, and the weights used will influence the answer obtained.

Additionally, use of age-standardised rates generates a 'hypothetical' estimate for the purposes of comparison across populations. However, it is likely that this will not reflect the true age/sex burden of the outcome actually being experienced in the study population. Use of age/sex-standardised rates for inequality comparisons means that the actual burden of inequality is not reflected. Thus such an approach can 'distort' the true age/sex burden by manipulating the crude rates according to some hypothetical standard population.

Further reading

Julious, S.A., Nicholl, J. and George, S. (2001) 'Why do we continue to use standardized mortality ratios for small area comparisons?', *Journal of Public Health Medicine*, vol 23, pp 40-6.

Silcocks, P.B.S., Jenner, D.A. and Reza, R. (2001) 'Life expectancy as a summary of mortality in a population: statistical considerations and suitability for use by health authorities', *Journal of Epidemiology and Community Health*, vol 55, pp 38-43.

See also: 4.11 Incidence; 4.14 Populations; 4.15 Prevalence; 4.17 Proportions

3.13 Theil Index and mean log deviation

The Theil Index and mean log deviation are examples of disproportionality measures of inequality (see **3.6 Measures of average disproportionality**). One class of disproportionality measures that is often favoured by economists is so-called measures of 'general entropy', first developed by Henri Theil (1967). The Theil Index (T) and mean log deviation (MLD) are both disproportionality measures of inequality that summarise differences as the natural logarithm of shares of health compared to shares of population. They may be written as follows:

$$T = \sum_{j=1}^{J} p_j r_j \ln r_j$$

$$MLD = \sum_{j=1}^{J} p_j - \ln r_j$$

where p_j is the proportion of the population in group j and r_j is the ratio of health in group j relative to the total rate, that is, $r_j = y_j / \mu$ where y_j is the prevalence of the outcomes in group j and μ is the total prevalence.

When the population of individuals is arranged into J groups, Theil showed that the equation above is the exact sum of two parts: between-group inequality and a weighted average of within-group inequality:

$$T = \sum_{j=1}^{J} p_j r_j \ln(r_j) + \sum_{j=1}^{J} p_j r_j T_j$$

where T_j is the inequality in health within group j. The within-group component (the second term on the right side of equation) is weighted by, in this case, group j's share of the total health, since $p_j \times r_j = y_j$ (where y_j is the *share* of total health) when the denominator for r_j is mean health for the total population. More importantly, the above decomposition also makes it clear that it is possible to calculate between-group inequality in health – the primary quantity of interest with respect to social inequalities in health – in the absence of data on each individual. The only data needed are the group proportions and the ratio of the group's health to the population average health. However, between-group health inequality may increase because total health inequality is increasing (that is, both between-group and within-group inequality are increasing simultaneously).

Strengths

The primary advantage of using measures like the Theil Index and the mean log deviation is that they are additively decomposable inequality measures. This means that it is possible to determine not just whether between-group inequality is increasing, but whether the share of total inequality that is due to inequality between groups is increasing or decreasing. Additionally, they can be applied to both rankable and un-rankable social groups.

Limitations

While this measure has very attractive qualities, the between-group/within-group decomposition requires continuous outcome data measurable in individuals, so it is not clear whether this can be applied to many relevant health outcomes, such as mortality, which are dichotomous. However, even for non-continuous outcomes, entropy indices can be used to calculate between-group inequalities in the absence of individual-level data. Additionally, these measures are quite unfamiliar to most researchers and stakeholders in the health inequalities field.

Example

Theil Index (T) and mean log deviation (MLD) applied to the change in social group inequality in health between 1990 and 2001					
Social group	Rate per 100,000 $[\mu_j]$	Population share $[p_j]$	Rate relative to total $[r_j]$	T $[p_j \times r_j \times \ln(r_j)]$	MLD $[p_j \times -\ln(r_j)]$
1990					
A	9.5	0.006	0.375	−0.0023	0.0062
B	14.5	0.026	0.570	−0.0084	0.0147
C	35.9	0.100	1.412	0.0486	−0.0344
D	24.7	0.868	0.970	−0.0255	0.0263
Total	25.5			0.0124	*0.0128*
2001					
A	10.4	0.009	0.541	−0.0029	0.0053
B	12.1	0.040	0.629	−0.0116	0.0184
C	30.0	0.109	1.559	0.0751	−0.0482
D	18.3	0.843	0.950	−0.0410	0.0431
Total	19.2			0.0198	*0.0186*

In this case both the Theil Index and the mean log deviation show increases in overall social group inequality in health.

References
Theil, H. (1967) *Economics and information theory*, Amsterdam: North Holland.

Further reading
Goesling, B. and Firebaugh G. (2004) 'The trend in international health inequality', *Population and Development Review*, vol 30, pp 131-46.

Hosseinpoor, A., van Doorslaer, E., Speybroeck, N., Naghavi, M., Mohammad, K., Majdzadeh, R., Delavar, B., Jamshidi, H. and Vega, J. (2006) 'Decomposing socioeconomic inequality in infant mortality in Iran', *International Journal of. Epidemiology*, vol 35, pp 1211-19.

Wagstaff, A. and van Doorslaer, E. (2004) 'Overall versus socioeconomic health inequality: a measurement framework and two empirical illustrations', *Health Economics*, vol 13, pp 297-301.

Zhang, Q. and Wang, Y. (2004) 'Socioeconomic inequality of obesity in the United States: do gender, age, and ethnicity matter?', *Social Science & Medicine*, vol 58, pp 1171-80.

See also: 3.6 Measures of average disproportionality

Part Four
Theoretical and methodological issues

4.1 Age-period cohort analysis (or effects)

One or a combination of age, period or cohort effects may drive changes in trends over time, for example, producing a widening or narrowing of socioeconomic differences in an outcome or leading to an increase or decrease in an outcome for one socioeconomic group alone.

Age effects mean that the change occurs in all individuals at a particular age irrespective of when they were born or the current time period. For example, an increase in socioeconomic differentials occurring at the age of retirement (irrespective of what time period is being examined or which birth cohort individuals were born in) would be described as an age effect.

A *cohort* is a group of people defined by a particular attribute (or set of attributes). In the context of age-period cohort effects, 'cohort' refers to birth cohort. Thus, the group (cohort) are defined by the period (usually the year) in which they were born.

Cohort analysis is the tabulation and analysis of data, such as morbidity and mortality rates or educational outcomes, in relation to the birth cohorts of the individuals concerned.

Cohort effect (also known as *generational effect*) refers to variations in health status that arise from the different causal factors to which each birth cohort in the population is exposed. Every birth cohort is exposed to different social and environmental circumstances that coincide with its life span. Because the meaning of socioeconomic measurements varies by birth cohorts (for example, a female who was born in 1910 obtaining a university degree is likely to have been from a different social stratum to a female born in 1975 obtaining a university degree) cohort effects are important to consider when examining the association of socioeconomic position (SEP) with health and other outcomes.

Some socioeconomic effects may be *birth cohort-specific*. For example, a recent cross-cohort study found that for British women born in the 1920s and 1930s childhood SEP was positively associated with hysterectomy rates (those from higher socioeconomic groups more likely to have a hysterectomy), for those born in the 1940s there was a weak inverse association and for those born in the 1950s a stronger inverse association (those from higher socioeconomic groups less likely to have a hysterectomy) (Cooper et al, 2005). This cohort effect may be related to the oldest generation having been brought up by parents who lived most of their lives prior to the introduction of the National Health Service.

Morbidity or mortality rates could vary because of changes in the way diseases are recognised and classified, changes in coding rules, changes in the incidence of disease, improvements in the effectiveness of treatment, and so on. These changes are likely to occur at specific periods of time and to affect different generations (birth cohorts) at the same time. These effects are known as *period effects*. For example, if the utilisation of a new effective treatment varies by socioeconomic group its introduction may result in a widening of socioeconomic inequalities compared to the time period before its introduction. If there is no age or generational effect on the utilisation then this change in inequalities is driven largely by a period effect.

Age-period cohort analyses

In reality socioeconomic differentials are dynamic and there is evidence that they change in both magnitude and direction over time and between geographical locations (Davey Smith and Lynch, 2004). It is clearly important to remember this and not to assume that in all circumstances, in all populations, at all time periods all health outcomes are worse in those from the lower socioeconomic groups (Vagero and Leinsalu, 2005).

It is likely that for many changes over time in socioeconomic inequalities age, cohort and period effects are relevant, but their relative importance may vary for different times and outcomes.

Age-period cohort analyses try to disentangle the influences operating over the individual's lifetime from those operating at a specific time on all generations. There is, however, an unresolved problem in trying to pin down the observed changes to one or the other of age, period or cohort effect because these are clearly not independent. Once two of the three are known the other is determined. If there is a linear change in an outcome over time it would be impossible to say if this were largely due to a period or cohort effect.

Several statistical regression models have been proposed to estimate the non-linear effects of period and cohort separately (Lee and Lin, 1995). These all make assumptions in order to produce unique parameter estimates, which need to be checked for biological plausibility.

References

Cooper, R., Lawlor, D.A., Hardy, R., Ebrahim, S., Leon, D.A., Wadsworth, M.E.J. and Kuh, D. (2005) 'Socioeconomic position across the life course and hysterectomy in three British cohorts: a cross-cohort comparative study', *British Journal of Obstetrics & Gynaecology*, vol 112, pp 1126-33.

Davey Smith, G. and Lynch. J. (2004) 'Life course approaches to socioeconomic differentials in health', in D. Kuh and Y. Ben-Shlomo (eds) *A life course approach to chronic disease epidemiology* (2nd edn), Oxford: Oxford University Press.

Lee, W.C. and Lin, R.S. (1995) 'Analysis of cancer rates using excess risk age-period-cohort models', *International Journal of Epidemiology*, vol 24, pp 671-7.

Vagero, D. and Leinsalu, M. (2005) 'Commentary: health inequalities and social dynamics in Europe', *BMJ*, vol 331, pp 186-7.

Further reading

Charlton, J. and Murphy, M. (1997) 'Monitoring health – data sources and methods', in J. Charlton and M. Murphy (eds) *The health of adult Britain: 1841-1994*, London: The Stationery Office, pp 2-16.

See also: 1.7 Life course socioeconomic position

4.2 Atomistic fallacy

The atomistic fallacy can occur when interpreting individual data and extrapolating to an ecological/area level. If individual-level data are used to investigate an association, that association may not hold at the aggregate or area level; to assume that it does is to invoke the atomistic (sometimes referred to as 'individualistic') fallacy. For example, a UK study of income and cerebrovascular disease mortality might find an inverse relationship (people with greater income being less likely to die from a stroke). However, it may be inappropriate to extrapolate this association to the international level; it is not necessarily the case that countries with the highest per capita income will have the lowest stroke mortality. The atomistic fallacy is a concept that may be contrasted with the much more widely known *ecological fallacy*. While the ecological fallacy highlights a potential problem with aggregate or area-level studies, the atomistic fallacy can occur with individual-level studies.

Problems related to the atomistic fallacy may also come into play if risk factors or influences beyond the individual are important but ignored. This is especially the case with measures of socioeconomic position (SEP). For example, an individual's social class, educational attainment and income may be used to study the relationship between SEP and some particular health outcome. It is possible that there is an additional effect of the SEP of the household, community or population in which that individual lives, which cannot simply be inferred from the individual's characteristics. If this contextual information is not collected, important or interesting information about the association between SEP and the health outcome may be missed. There is ongoing debate about the relative importance of socioeconomic 'context' and 'composition', and multilevel analysis techniques have been proposed as one means of investigating these issues.

Further reading

Diez-Roux, A.V. (1998) 'Bringing context back into epidemiology: variables and fallacies in multilevel analysis', *American Journal of Public Health*, vol 88, no 2, pp 216-22.

Leyland, A.H. and Groenewegen, P.P. (2003) 'Multilevel modelling and public health policy', *Scandinavian Journal of Public Health*, vol 31, no 4, pp 267-74.

Schwartz, S. (1994) 'The fallacy of the ecological fallacy: the potential misuse of a concept and the consequences', *American Journal of Public Health*, vol 84, no 5, pp 819-24.

See also: 4.8 Ecological fallacy

4.3 Bar charts

Bar charts (also known as bar graphs) are used to present discrete (categorical) data. Each observation can fall into only one category (for example, each social group). Frequencies for each group of observations are represented by the heights of the corresponding bars.

Examples

The first figure shows a bar graph depicting life expectancy from birth for different birth cohorts (see **4.1 Age-period cohort analysis (or effects)**) for women and men born in England and Wales in different years. This graph shows that for each birth cohort, life expectancy from birth is greater for women than men. It also shows that life expectancy has increased for both men and women over time, with the fastest increases during the first half of the 20th century.

Life expectancy from birth in England and Wales, 1840s-1990s

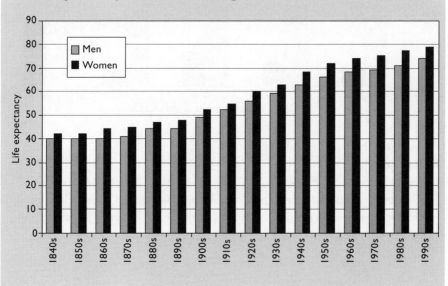

The second figure shows a bar graph illustrating the relationship between father's occupational social class at birth on cardiovascular disease (coronary heart disease [CHD] and stroke) among middle-aged adults who were born in Aberdeen, Scotland, in the 1950s (Lawlor et al, 2006). The graph shows that incidence of cardiovascular disease is higher when father's social class at birth is lower, and this is particularly so for social class V.

Incidence of cardiovascular disease by father's social class in middle-aged adults in Aberdeen, Scotland in the 1950s

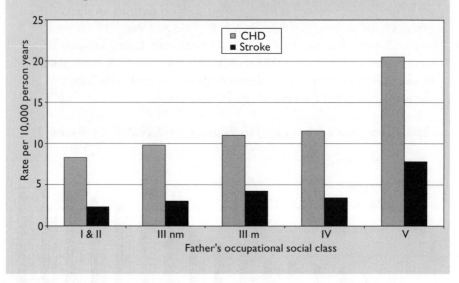

References

Lawlor, D., Ronalds, G., Macintyre, S., Clark, H. and Leon, D.A. (2006) 'Family socioeconomic position at birth predicts future cardiovascular disease risk: findings from the Aberdeen Children of the 1950s Cohort Study', *American Journal of Public Health*, vol 96, pp 1271-7.

4.4 Box and whisker plots

Box and whisker plots are a graphical way of comparing the distribution of a
continuous outcome variable in two or more exposure groups. The minimum
and maximum values of the outcome variable are indicated by the extremities
(or 'whiskers') of the diagram while the horizontal lines at the top and bottom
of the 'box' represent the upper and lower quartiles (25th and 75th percentiles
respectively). Thus, the middle 50% of the distribution is contained in the box.
The horizontal line inside the box represents the median (50th percentile) of
the outcome variable.

Example

The figure shows a box and whisker plot of waist circumference by adult
occupational social class among British women aged 60-79 years. This
shows, for example, that the median waist circumference for women
with non-manual jobs is around 825mm, while for women with manual
jobs it is around 850mm. The 'boxes' and 'whiskers' show how the waist
circumference measurements are distributed around the median for each
group.

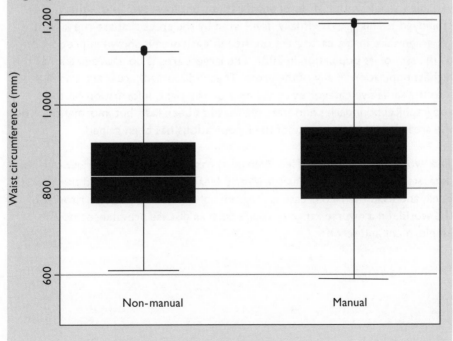

4.5 Cartograms

A cartogram is an alternative method of representing geographical data (such as mortality rates for wards, or populations of local authority areas) to that used in conventional maps. Instead of representing the physical boundaries of areas, cartograms show areas defined in proportion to some variable of interest. There are various types of cartogram; a common form is the Dorling cartogram that uses a uniform shape, such as a circle or hexagon, to represent each area. The size of the circle or hexagon (or collection of hexagons) relates to the size of the population (or variable) being represented. These areas can then be shaded to represent the values of another variable. The cartogram is useful because it allows us to see the areas that are physically small, but that have large populations (cities). At the same time it de-emphasises areas that are geographically large but whose populations are relatively small; such areas can visually dominate a traditional map.

In the example below the traditional map on the right shows the actual boundaries of 142 areas across the UK (counties, unitary authorities, former metropolitan authorities, council areas [in Scotland], and Northern Ireland as a whole). The areas are shaded by five categories according to another variable (people with high-level qualifications but low-level jobs – the 'under-employed'). This map is visually dominated by the areas that are the largest geographically. In the cartogram on the left each area is shown in proportion to the size of its population in 2001. The largest area is London since it has the highest population of any of the areas. These (distorted) areas are also shaded into the same five categories as the map on the right. Information on the geographical boundaries and sizes of areas has been lost, but information about the areas in terms of the size of their populations has been gained.

The Worldmapper project (see Weblinks) has collated a wide variety of global datasets from sources such as the World Health Organization and the World Bank, and used them to create cartograms of all countries and territories of the world, on a diverse range of topics such as disease prevalence, income, employment and so on.

Strengths

The cartogram is a much 'fairer' representation of social phenomena – each person (or other unit of interest) is effectively given the same amount of space on the map. On a conventional map, it is often the case that the largest areas have the smallest populations, and vice versa.

Limitations

The cartogram presents the user with an unfamiliar map that takes some effort to read, and may not allow intuitive identification of places of interest. In some circumstances, the geographical location is important, and a cartogram is inappropriate.

Example

Variation in percentage of people with high-level qualifications working in the lowest three socioeconomic classes across 142 areas of the UK

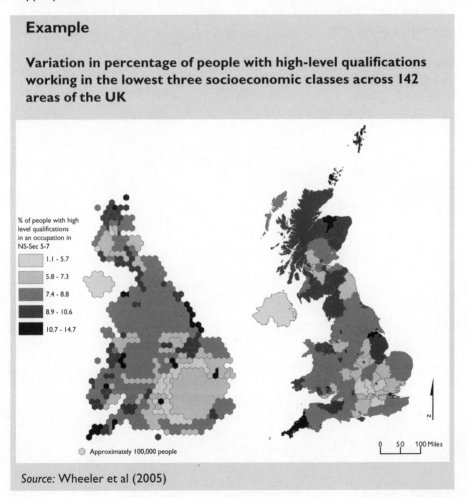

% of people with high level qualifications in an occupation in NS-Sec 5-7

- 1.1 - 5.7
- 5.8 - 7.3
- 7.4 - 8.8
- 8.9 - 10.6
- 10.7 - 14.7

Approximately 100,000 people

0   50   100 Miles

Source: Wheeler et al (2005)

References

Wheeler, B., Shaw, M., Mitchell, R. and Dorling, D. (2005) *Life in Britain: Using millennial Census data to understand poverty, inequality and place*, Bristol: The Policy Press (www. shef.ac.uk/sasi/research/life_in_britain.htm) [A pack of 10 reports, a technical, summary and five posters produced for the Joseph Rowntree Foundation].

Further reading

Dorling, D. and Fairburn, D. (1997) *Mapping: Ways of representing the world*, Harlow: Addison Wesley Longman.

Thomas, B. and Dorling, D. (2004) *People and places: A 2001 census atlas of the UK*, Bristol: The Policy Press.

Weblinks

A series of global cartograms of various data from the UN, World Bank and so on: www.worldmapper.org

See also: 2.23 National Statistics Socioeconomic Classification (NS-SEC); 4.6 Choropleth maps; 4.10 Geographic information systems (GIS)

4.6 Choropleth maps

A choropleth map shows geographical patterns and distributions by using different symbols – usually different colours or shading – for areas (or polygons) on a map that represent quantitative data that has been classed in some way. The areas marked can represent any number of geographical units, such as countries, regions, counties, local authorities or electoral wards. For example, the map below shows counties, unitary authorities and similar areas shaded by the percentage of the population with both poor health and limiting long-term illness from the 2001 Census.

Choropleth maps are the most familiar form of the representation of geographical data, and are a highly effective means of communication. The main drawback of this type of map is that for administrative geographies the largest administrative units tend to be sparsely populated rural units, while the smallest tend to be densely populated urban areas. This means that the map emphasises the areas in which few people live while at the same time de-emphasising the areas containing most of the population. Cartograms (see **4.5**) are an alternative form of mapping that addresses this issue.

Discussion point

One of the most important things to look at with a choropleth map is how the data have been classified to produce the different categories. In the example map, values range from 3.5% to 16.5%, and these have been divided up into five categories, each containing a fifth of the areas (quintiles). However, the data could have been classified in many different ways. How might the map look with just four categories? Or seven? How would it look if the categories were of equal size, such as 1%-5%, 5%-10%, 10%-15%, 15%-20%? It is not possible to tell without having the data that were used to make the map.

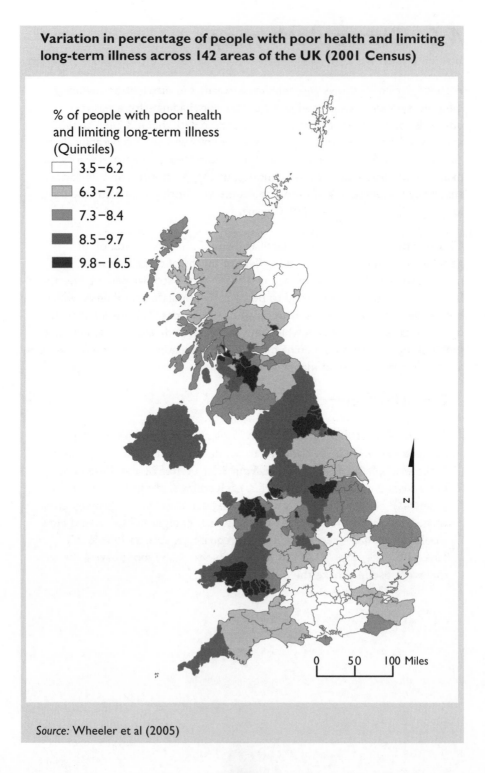

Variation in percentage of people with poor health and limiting long-term illness across 142 areas of the UK (2001 Census)

% of people with poor health and limiting long-term illness (Quintiles)

- 3.5–6.2
- 6.3–7.2
- 7.3–8.4
- 8.5–9.7
- 9.8–16.5

0   50   100 Miles

Source: Wheeler et al (2005)

References

Wheeler, B., Shaw, M., Mitchell, R. and Dorling, D. (2005) *Life in Britain: Using millennial Census data to understand poverty, inequality and place*, Bristol: The Policy Press (www. shef.ac.uk/sasi/research/life_in_britain.htm) [A pack of 10 reports, a technical, summary and five posters produced for the Joseph Rowntree Foundation].

Further reading

Dorling, D. and Fairburn, D. (1997) *Mapping: Ways of representing the world*, Harlow: Addison Wesley Longman.

Monmonier, M. (1996) *How to lie with maps*, Chicago, IL: University of Chicago Press.

Thomas, B. and Dorling, D. (2004) *People and places: A 2001 census atlas of the UK*, Bristol: The Policy Press.

See also: 4.5 Cartogram; 4.10 Geographic information systems (GIS)

4.7 Correlation coefficients

The correlation coefficient is a simple summary measure of the strength of the linear association between two continuous variables. The easiest way to understand the correlation coefficient is to relate it to a **scatter plot** (see **4.18**), such as those in the figure below. When two variables, x and y, are plotted on this kind of graph, the correlation coefficient tells you how closely the points lie to a diagonal straight line.

The coefficient can take on a value between −1 and +1. A value of +1 indicates a perfect positive relationship – as one variable increases, the other also does so in direct proportion. A perfect negative (or inverse) relationship is indicated by −1; as one increases, the other decreases in direct proportion. A value of 0 means that there is no (linear) relationship between the two variables. As a statistical measure, correlation coefficients have a lot of statistical power, which means that even with very weak correlations p-values tend to be small, suggesting 'statistical significance'. Thus it is important to concentrate on the actual value of the correlation coefficient. In general coefficients greater than 0.6 (or less than −0.6) are considered strong, those from 0.4 to 0.6 (−0.4 to −0.6) modest and those between −0.4 and 0.4 are considered weak.

Strengths

The correlation coefficient is a fairly simple and commonly used measure, and combined with a scatter plot can give a quick idea of the nature of the relationship between two variables.

Limitations

This statistic does not tell you anything about how much y increases when x increases (the slope of the line). For example, if we had data for local authorities on mortality rates and unemployment rates, we might get a reasonably strong correlation of, say, +0.7. This tells us that the mortality rate tends to be higher in areas with higher unemployment, but not how much higher. The same correlation coefficient could result from relationships where a 1% increase in unemployment was associated with an increase of 1 death per 100,000, or 5 deaths per 100,000, or 600 deaths per 100,000.

The statistic also assumes that the relationship between the two variables can be described by a straight line – if x and y are associated, but in a non-linear fashion – the correlation coefficient may be misleading (see the last graph in the figure).

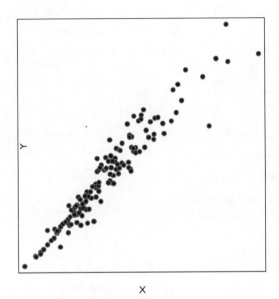

Very strong positive correlation. As x increases, y increases

Correlation coefficient = 0.96

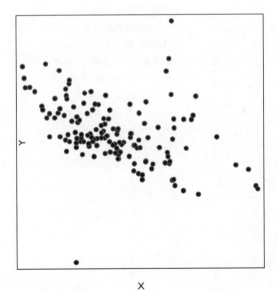

Weak or moderate negative correlation – as x increases, y decreases, but the points do not lie in a very tight line

Correlation coefficient = −0.41

Note that the coefficient can be affected by outliers – removing the two data points with the highest and lowest values of y here gives a stronger coefficient of −0.53

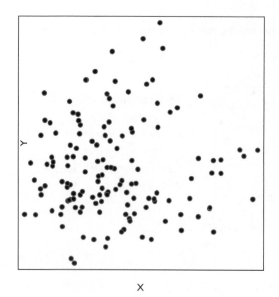

No discernible association between x and y

Correlation coefficient = 0.03

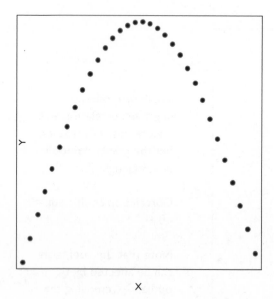

An extreme example of how a correlation coefficient can be misleading. There is obviously an extremely strong relationship between x and y, but it is not linear. The correlation coefficient here is 0.05, indicating no strong association (in fact y=Sin(x))

See also: 4.18 Scatter plots

4.8 Ecological fallacy

The ecological fallacy can occur when interpreting ecological (spatial, area-level or aggregate) data. It relates to doing an analysis at one level, and then inferring that finding to another level. Most usually, the term is used to refer to assuming that the relationships found between variables at an area level hold for the relationship between those variables at the individual level.

A classic example can be drawn from Robinson (1950). Robinson looked at literacy (in American-English) rates and the proportion of people who were foreign-born for 48 states of the US, finding that in states with a higher proportion of foreign-born people literacy rates were higher (correlation coefficient of 0.53). This might imply that foreign-born individuals were more likely to be literate in American-English than the native-born – but to assume that this was the case at the individual level would be to fall foul of the ecological fallacy. In this case, at the individual level the relationship between foreign birth and American-English literacy was actually negative (correlation coefficient of −0.11). The correlation found at the area level is due to the fact foreign-born people were more likely to live in states where the native-born had relatively high levels of literacy.

Another example would be to assume, if in higher income countries it was found that mortality rates from road traffic accidents were higher than in poorer countries, that *within* any of those countries people with higher incomes would have higher rates of road traffic accident mortality than less well-off people.

Any assumptions made about individuals based on aggregate data are vulnerable to the ecological fallacy. However, that does not mean that it is not useful to compare the characteristics of areas, just that ecological associations are unreliable indicators of individual associations.

Discussion point

Are areas poor?

The idea of 'poverty' is not simply descriptive; it is a moral term, implying an evaluation of circumstances (Piachaud, 1981). To argue that an area is 'poor' is not simply to say that there are not many resources, but that there is a problem. That has to be based in the position that the area itself can be an appropriate focus for moral concern. Like many moral positions, this does not lend itself easily to argument; ultimately one either accepts it or one does not.

The central objection to describing an area as 'poor' is individualistic: that there is no such thing as an area, only the people who make it up. It is not, then, areas which have problems or low incomes, but the people who live in them. It would still follow that the area will have a higher concentration of poor people than elsewhere; it will have a variety of social problems; and the conditions of poor people are likely to be worse than if the same people lived elsewhere. Even from an individualistic perspective, then, there is still a case for considering the impact of location on poverty.

The case for shifting the focus of attention to the area becomes markedly stronger when attention moves to people who are not themselves poor. Living in a poor area can act to their detriment. It happens, for example, through the lack of community resources, the increased competition for places in the labour market, and the effect of stigmatisation on command over resources. Further, people who live in such areas are less secure than others. The fear of crime is directly associated with perceptions of the physical deterioration of an area (Painter, 1992, p 182), but the problems are not simply a matter of perception. People who are on higher incomes in lower income areas have greater vulnerability to crime than people elsewhere, including burglary, robbery, motor vehicle theft and vandalism (Evans, 1992, pp 42-6). These people are not likely to be made poor in consequence – that would happen only if the effect of living in the area was to bring their level of resources down sufficiently to consider them as deprived – but anyone in this position has lower resources, other things being equal, than others who have desirable, well-maintained environments.

Source: Spicker (2001)

References

Evans, D. (1992) 'Left realism and the spatial study of crime', in D. Evans, N. Fyfe and D. Herbert (eds) *Crime, policing and place: Essays in environmental criminology*, London: Routledge.

Painter, K. (1992) 'Different worlds', in D. Evans, N. Fyfe and D. Herbert (eds) *Crime, policing and place: Essays in environmental criminology*, London: Routledge.

Piachaud, D. (1981) 'Peter Townsend and the Holy Grail', *New Society*, 10 September, pp 419-21.

Robinson, W. (1950) 'Ecological correlations and the behavior of individuals', *American Sociological Review*, vol 15, pp 351-7.

Spicker, P. (2001) 'Poor areas and the "ecological fallacy"', *Radical Statistics*, vol 76 (www.radstats.org.uk).

Further reading

Macintyre, S., Maciver, S. and Sooman, A. (1993) 'Area, class and health: should we be focusing on places or people?', *Journal of Social Policy*, vol 22, no 2, pp 213-34.

Schwartz, S. (1994) 'The fallacy of the ecological fallacy: the potential misuses of a concept and the consequences', *American Journal of Public Heath*, vol 84, no 5, pp 819-24.

See also: 4.2 Atomistic fallacy

4.9 Funnel plots

Funnel plots are graphs used in meta-analyses that help to identify whether publication bias (or some other bias) might be operating. They are also used in the public health context to look at variation in rates and so on (see below).

A meta-analysis compares and pools the results of a number of studies on the same issue to see if there is a consistent pattern of results, and to obtain a pooled estimate of the effect using the combined power of all of the studies. These studies can be prone to 'publication bias'. For a meta-analysis of a particular risk–outcome relationship using published study results, if only those studies producing a positive, statistically significant result are published, and studies producing a negative or statistically insignificant result are not, the meta-analysis may be affected by publication bias. This bias in publication may be due to non-significant or 'uninteresting' studies not being written up by the investigators, or through rejection from journals. The funnel plot cannot confirm that publication bias is present, only that some sort of bias may be operating or that there may be other quality issues with one or more of the studies.

The funnel plot is a **scatter plot**, plotting the effect estimate (such as risk ratio, odds ratio or mean difference) from each study on the x-axis, and some measure of the precision (usually the standard error of the effect estimate, but could be sample size or some other precision measure) of the study along the y-axis. The example illustrates these plots, and how they might identify a problem with the meta-analysis.

Example

Figure A shows a hypothetical funnel plot from a meta-analysis where the effect estimate from each study is a risk ratio (RR), and the measure of precision for each RR is its standard error. The RR and its standard error are plotted against each other (log scales are used here since this is a ratio measure, so the distance on the RR scale between 0.01 and 0.1 is the same as that between 1 and 10). The dashed line indicates the pooled RR, found from combining the data from all of the studies in the meta-analysis. A lower standard error indicates greater precision, so we would expect to see studies with lower standard error falling closer to the pooled estimate.

The plot is roughly symmetrical, producing the 'inverted funnel' shape from which the graph name is derived. Studies with low precision (high standard error) appear to be just as likely to be over-estimates as they are under-estimates (compared to the pooled estimate), which is reassuring with regard to publication bias.

Figure A: Hypothetical funnel plot

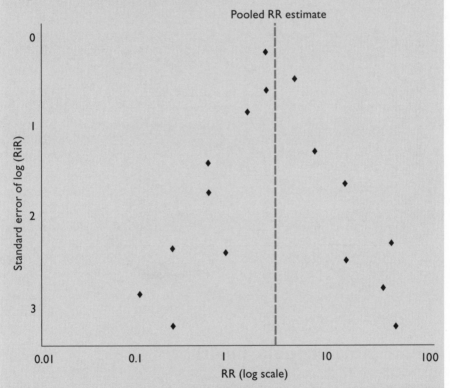

The plot in Figure B has a distinctly asymmetrical shape – it appears that effect estimates from low-precision studies are all much larger than those from more precise studies. This might suggest that publication bias, or some other systematic error, could be in operation, and the results of the meta-analysis may therefore be worthy of further investigation.

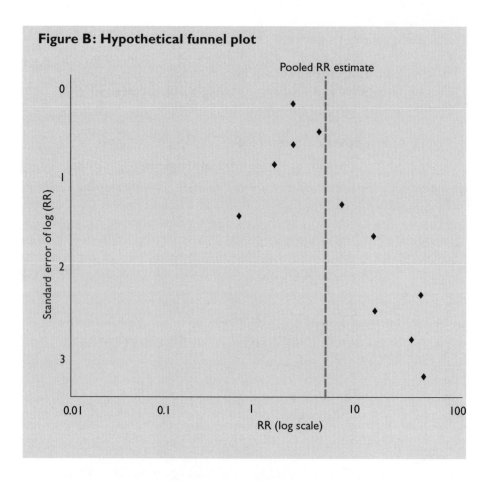

Figure B: Hypothetical funnel plot

Funnel plots in public health

Very similar funnel plots are used in the public health context to investigate and visualise variations in disease and death rates across different areas and so on. These are plotted in a similar manner, with a measure of precision on one axis (often population size), and the measure of interest (such as mortality rate) on the other. Additionally, 'control limits' are usually plotted onto the chart, which allow easy recognition of those data points falling above or below values that might be expected. These points can then be investigated further.

Example

The funnel plot here shows obesity (BMI>30) prevalence for each Government Office Region of England in 2001 based on sample surveys. The plot shows sample size (measure of precision) against obesity prevalence for each region. It also shows the England average, and 95% control limits, which enables the regions with unusually high and low prevalence to be highlighted and identified.

Figure C: Example of a public health funnel plot: obesity prevalence for the English regions

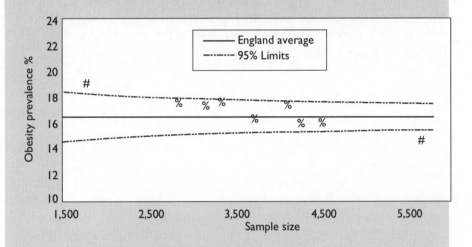

Adapted from: APHO (Association of Public Health Observatories) (2003) 'Indications of public health in the English Regions', vol 1, no 1 (www.pho.org.uk/documents/indicators.pdf)

Further Reading

Egger, M., Davey Smith, G., Schneider, M. and Minder, C. (1997) 'Bias in meta-analysis detected by a simple, graphical test', *BMJ*, vol 315, no 7109, pp 629-34.

Weblinks

Cochrane Collaboration tutorial on funnel plots:
www.cochrane-net.org/openlearning/HTML/mod15-3.htm
Eastern Region Public Health Observatory Funnel Plot Tools
www.erpho.org.uk/topics/tools/funnel.aspx

4.10 Geographic information systems (GIS)

A geographical information system (GIS) is a system for capturing, storing, checking, integrating, manipulating, analysing and displaying quantitative (and sometimes qualitative) data that are spatially referenced. For example, a GIS might store information on: the location of road traffic collisions, Accident and Emergency departments at hospitals, or pubs; the road network and the type of roads; and the characteristics of the population at a small area level derived from census data (for example, age/sex structure, car ownership, deprivation). The relationships between these factors could then be explored. There is a range of GIS software packages available. One of the most common uses of GIS is for producing maps.

Variation in unemployment rates across the 142 areas of the UK (2001)

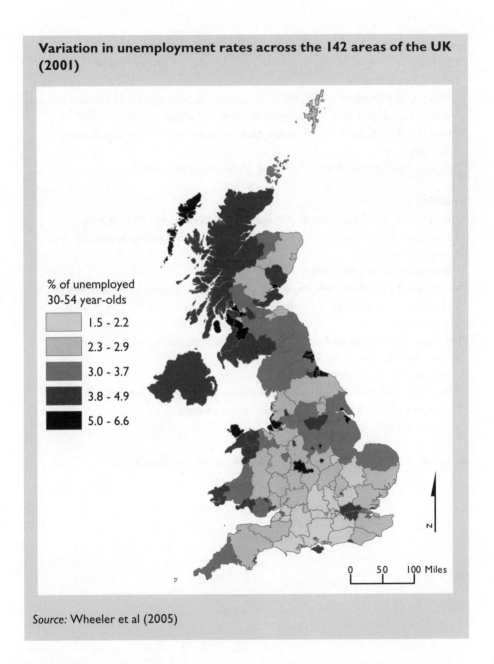

% of unemployed
30-54 year-olds

- 1.5 - 2.2
- 2.3 - 2.9
- 3.0 - 3.7
- 3.8 - 4.9
- 5.0 - 6.6

0   50   100 Miles

Source: Wheeler et al (2005)

References

Wheeler, B., Shaw, M., Mitchell, R. and Dorling, D. (2005) *Life in Britain: Using millennial Census data to understand poverty, inequality and place*, Bristol: The Policy Press (www. shef.ac.uk/sasi/research/life_in_britain.htm) [A pack of 10 reports, a technical, summary and five posters produced for the Joseph Rowntree Foundation].

Further reading

BCS (British Cartographic Society) (1991) *Cartography and geographic information systems*, London: BCS.

Gordon, A. and Womersley, J. (1997) 'The use of mapping in public health and planning health services', *Journal of Public Health Medicine*, vol 19, pp 139-47.

Martin, D. (1996) *Geographic information systems: Socioeconomic applications*, London: Routledge.

The Cartographic Journal, Maney Publishing, three issues per year.

Weblinks

Home page for GIS Research UK (GISRUK), the UK's national GIS research conference, established in 1993. GISRUK conferences are primarily aimed at the academic community:

www.geo.ed.ac.uk/gisruk/gisruk.html

Website run by a private company in the US, ESRI (Environmental Systems Research Institute), which produces ArcInfo and other software:

www.gis.com

MAPresso is a free Java applet for unclassed choropleth maps and cartograms:

www.mapresso.com

Association for Geographic Information:

"The Mission of the AGI is to maximise the use of geographic information (GI) for the benefit of the citizen, good governance and commerce":

www.agi.org.uk

See also: 4.5 Cartograms; 4.6 Choropleth maps; 4.8 Ecological fallacy

4.11 Incidence

Incidence refers to the number of new events (such as new cases of disease, people starting to smoke) in a defined population within a specified period of time. Incidence refers to new cases occurring in a specified time period, which that distinguishes it from prevalence, which counts the total number of events (old and new) in a time period. For example, the number of newly diagnosed cases of lung cancer reported to a cancer registry in a month is a measure of incidence. The number of people living with lung cancer at a specific point in time (whenever diagnosed/reported) is a measure of prevalence.

Incidence rate: the rate at which new events occur in a population. The numerator is the number of new events that occur in a defined population; the denominator is the population at risk of experiencing the event during this period, sometimes expressed as 'person-time'.

Incidence rate ratio: the incidence rate in the exposed group divided by the incidence rate in the unexposed group. Often referred to as the 'rate ratio' (see 3.9 **Relative differences**).

Example

The table below shows the incidence rate and rate ratio of coronary heart disease (CHD) occurring in the first four years of follow-up of the British Women's Heart and Health Study among participants who were free of heart disease at baseline. A comparison is made between those women who were living in publicly funded housing (council housing) at baseline and women living in privately owned or rented housing.

	Number with incident case of CHD	Person years at risk	Incidence rate (95% confidence interval) per 1,000	Incidence rate ratio
Private housing	143	15,314.3	9.34 (7.93, 11.00)	1
Public housing	40	2,373.0	16.86 (12.36, 22.98)	1.78 (1.25, 2.53)

Since incidence is concerned with new events a prospective study design (with long-term follow-up) is necessary to estimate incidence. Such prospective studies allow for causal inferences to be made with more confidence than cross-sectional studies because the exposure (housing type in the above example) is clearly measured before the disease occurrence. In the above example new CHD cases occurred during the four years following collection of housing data, and all women with heart disease at the baseline were excluded.

See also: 4.14 Populations; 4.15 Prevalence

4.12 Line graphs

In research into socioeconomic inequalities, line graphs are commonly used to demonstrate trends over time among different socioeconomic groups for various outcomes, such as disease or other health-related outcomes. They are a simple and comprehensible visual tool for this purpose.

Example

Line graphs were used in a study relating trends over time in smoking prevalence by social class to trends in all-cause mortality (Lawlor et al, 2003). The first figure shows smoking prevalence by social class in UK men from 1948-99. There was very little socioeconomic differential in smoking prevalence in the late 1940s, but more marked declines in prevalence among the highest socioeconomic group (social class I, professionals) compared to the lowest group (V, unskilled manual workers) resulted in marked differentials from the 1960s onwards. These were exacerbated by a levelling out of the decline in the lowest groups from 1980 with continued declines from this time in higher groups.

Smoking prevalence among UK men 16 years and older, by social class (1948-99)

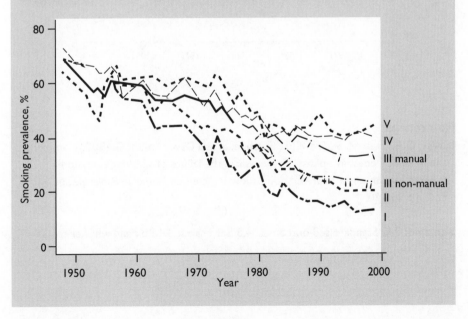

The second figure shows age-standardised all-cause mortality rates in UK men by social class from 1931-91. This shows that socioeconomic differentials in mortality were apparent from 1931 and began to widen particularly from 1951, some 10 years before the differentials in smoking behaviour. The authors concluded that the better life chances among those from the higher socioeconomic groups would have been likely to influence their rapid decline in smoking once knowledge of its detrimental effects became widely known and that, by contrast, persistent smoking among the most deprived members of society may represent a rational response to their life chances informed by a lay epidemiology.

Age-standardised all-cause mortality rate, men from England and Wales aged 20-64 years, by social class (1931-91)

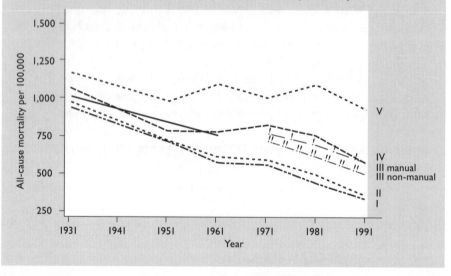

References

Lawlor, D.A., Frankel, S., Shaw, M., Ebrahim, S. and Davey Smith, G. (2003) 'Smoking and ill-health: does lay epidemiology explain the failure of smoking cessation programmes amongst deprived populations?', *American Journal of Public Health*, vol 93, no 2, pp 266-70.

See also: 3.12 Standardised outcomes; 4.3 Bar charts; 4.4 Box and whisker plots

4.13 Percentages

A percentage is a rate or proportion 'per cent', that is, converted to a denominator of 100 (cent). Prevalences are often presented as percentages. For example, if there are 600 men in social class V and 100 of these smoke, the percentage who smoke is 100/600 x 100 = 16.67%. A percentage can only take values of 0-100. For example, if no one in a particular social grouped smoked the percentage of smokers would be 0%; if all of them smoked it would be 100%. To convert a proportion to a percentage, multiply by 100, for example a proportion of 0.34 equates to 34%.

See also: 4.15 Prevalence; 4.17 Proportions

4.14 Populations

In social science, epidemiology and public health research, the term 'population' usually refers to the group of individuals being studied – the study population. Using a sample from that population, inferences are made about that population. A population is defined by a given set of attributes that may include geography but can also include other characteristics such as gender, age, ethnicity or social group. If a research question is concerned with socioeconomic inequalities among middle-aged Afro-Caribbean women who live in Europe, then the study population is all middle-aged (this should ideally be specified, for example, aged 40-55 years) Afro-Caribbean women who live in Europe. It is unlikely that any study will be able to collect data on all members of this population and so a random sample is sought from the population. It is important that the sample is random (meaning that every member of the population has the same chance of being in the study) otherwise the results from the study may not accurately reflect inequalities in the study population. In practice, however, samples are unlikely to be truly random, as often only certain types of individuals agree to participate. The extent of this selection process is important to consider in interpreting the results. If the sample is relatively random, the results from a selected study sample are generalisable to the population of this study, but one cannot assume that they are generalisable to another population (for example, middle-aged Caucasian men).

Populations can also be defined by time, for example, the populations of Britain in 1990, 1995 and 2000. Results derived from a study based on a sample of a population at one point in time may not be the same as those drawn from a sample of a population at a different time period. For example, the meaning of, and therefore likely effect of, educational attainment among westernised women in the 1920s is likely to be different from that of similar women in the 1990s.

See also: 3.12 Standardised outcomes

4.15 Prevalence

Prevalence relates to the total number of individuals who have a disease (or other attribute) in a given population at a particular time or during a particular time period. Prevalence is a proportion or a percentage, not a rate; a unit of time is not in the denominator. Prevalence is often expressed as a percentage. For example, if a baseline survey is conducted and questions are asked about smoking and occupation one can calculate the prevalence of current smoking (number of current smokers in social class/total number of individuals in social class) and ever smoking by social class (number of ever smokers in social class/total number of individuals in social class).

The prevalence is affected both by incidence (the number of new events occurring over a time period, such as people taking up smoking), recovery (or change in status, such as those giving up smoking) and mortality. For example, the prevalence of a condition may be low even with a high incidence if there is either a rapid recovery from the condition or rapid death from it. Conversely a condition with a relatively low incidence and that is not reversible, but does not lead to rapid death, will have a high prevalence.

Lifetime prevalence: the total number of people known to have had the disease (or other event of interest) for at least part of their lives divided by the total population at risk.

Period prevalence: the total number of people known to have had the disease (or other event of interest) at any time in a specified period (for example, 1995-2000) divided by the population at risk during that period.

Point prevalence: the total number of people with the disease (or other event of interest) at a specified point in time (for example, 1 March 2000) divided by the population at risk at that point.

Example

The table shows the prevalence of current and ever smoking among participants in the British Women's Heart and Health Study by adult social class at the time of the baseline survey (2000) for that study.

Prevalence of current and ever smoking by social class among British women aged 60-79 years in 2000

Social class	Total number in each social class	Number current smokers	Prevalence current smokers (%)	Number ever smokers	Prevalence ever smokers (%)
I professional	325	24	7.4	119	36.6
II	824	77	9.3	340	41.3
III non-manual	678	63	9.3	290	42.8
III manual	1,043	132	12.7	472	45.3
IV	538	61	11.3	235	43.7
V unskilled manual	859	138	16.1	440	51.2

Prevalence is a common method of measuring outcomes in cross-sectional and case control studies. These studies are unable to determine causality because the timing of exposure in relation to outcome is unclear. This is evident in the example from the cross-sectional study among British women. Although women from lower social classes are more likely to be current or ever smokers compared to those from higher social classes we do not know from this study whether social class leads to someone becoming a smoker or whether being a smoker influences one's job opportunities and therefore occupational-based social class.

See also: 4.11 Incidence; 4.13 Percentages; 4.17 Proportions

4.16 Proportional mortality ratio (PMR)

The proportional mortality ratio (PMR) is often used to calculate occupational mortality rates where denominator data are lacking, that is, when the population numbers in each subgroup are not available. This measure has been frequently used in the British Registrar General's Decennial Supplements. The proportion of observed deaths from a specific cause are divided by the proportion of deaths expected from that condition in a standard population, expressed either on an age-specific basis or after age adjustment. It does not require data on the age composition of the population, but only on the age composition of the deaths.

A PMR of 100 for a particular group indicates that there is no difference in the proportion of deaths from that particular cause compared to the standard population, whereas a PMR of 50 indicates that only half of the proportion of deaths from that cause that were expected were observed. A PMR of 200 on the other hand indicates that twice as many deaths occurred in the study group compared to the standard population.

Strengths

The PMR can be particularly appropriate for occupational epidemiology, and can be calculated where data on the age composition of the population is lacking.

Limitations

As well as an excess of deaths from the particular cause being examined, a high PMR can be the result of a low number of deaths from other causes. A low PMR could therefore indicate an excess of deaths from other causes or a low proportion of deaths from the cause being studied.

Example

In a study by Stark et al (2006) PMRs were calculated for deaths from suicide among men for occupational groups. In this case they calculated PMRs with 95% confidence intervals for two age groups (16-45 and 46-64) for those occupational categories with 10 or more deaths. The table shows occupations with significantly high and low PMRs for the younger of the two age groups.

Suicide and undetermined intent deaths, highest and lowest occupational PMRs with confidence intervals for men aged 16-45 years

	Number of deaths	PMR	Lower 95% confidence interval	Upper 95% confidence interval
Highest occupational PMRs				
Counter hands, assistants	16	195	112	316
Medical practitioners	26	180	118	265
Hotel porters	20	165	101	254
Forestry workers	40	163	116	221
Hospital, ward orderlies	22	163	102	247
Gardeners, groundsmen	126	146	122	173
Students at university/college	233	143	126	163
Security guards and officers, patrolmen, watchmen	81	137	110	170
Chefs, cooks	195	126	103	154
Building and civil engineering labourers	159	119	102	139
Labourers and unskilled workers not elsewhere classified	644	117	108	126
Lowest occupational PMRs				
Production, works and maintenance managers, works foremen	14	50	27	84
Office managers not elsewhere classified	14	54	30	91
Metal working production fitters and fitters/machinists	104	79	65	95
Machine tool operators	58	74	58	96
Electricians, electrical maintenance fitters	85	79	64	97
Drivers of road goods vehicles	157	83	71	97

Source: Adapted from Stark et al (2006)

Reference

Stark, C., Belbin, A., Hopkins, P., Gibbs, D., Hay, A. and Gunnell, D. (2006) 'Male suicide and occupation in Scotland', *Health Statistics Quarterly*, vol 29, pp 26-9.

See also: 3.12 Standardised outcomes

4.17 Proportions

A proportion is a portion or part in its relation to the whole. For example, if there are 600 men in social class V and 100 of these smoke, the proportion who smoke is 100/600 = 0.167. A proportion can only take values between 0 and 1. For example, if no one in a particular social group smoked the proportion of smokers would be 0; if all of them smoked it would be 1. To convert a percentage to a proportion, divide by 100, for example 34% equates to the proportion 0.34.

See also: 4.13 Percentages; 4.15 Prevalence

4.18 Scatter plots

A scatter plot is a graphical method of displaying the distribution of two continuous variables in relation to each other. The values for one variable are measured on the horizontal (x) axis and the values for the other on the vertical (y) axis. Values can be for individuals (in studies based on individuals) or can plot the means of variables from groups of individuals (for example, as used in ecological studies). Scatter plots are often presented showing the best line of fit that represents the linear relationship between the two variables obtained from a linear regression model. Scatter plots allow the range and distribution of values for two measures, and the relationship between them, to be quickly assessed. They are simple to understand but convey a lot of information. Unusual results can be identified, such as an area with a high level of poverty but a low level of mortality.

Example

The two figures below represent the linear relationship between body mass index (BMI) (a measure of general adiposity) and waist:hip ratio (a measure of central adiposity) among British women in manual (top figure) and non-manual (bottom figure) social classes. These show similar positive linear associations between these two measurements (although on average women from manual social classes have higher BMI and waist: hip ratios compared with those from non-manual classes).

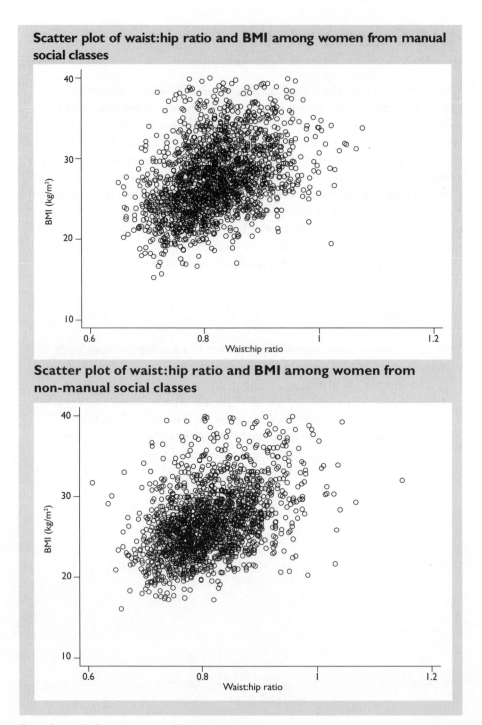

Scatter plot of waist:hip ratio and BMI among women from manual social classes

Scatter plot of waist:hip ratio and BMI among women from non-manual social classes

See also: 4.7 Correlation coefficients